All My Brother's Fingers and Toes

By Marlene E. Weiss

A story about what a mother's love can do

CHAPTER 1
Book Signing Party

It is Monday October 16, 2000, nine days after my fiftieth birthday, and I just got the best present ever. I am picking my mother up and taking her to her book-signing party in Naples, Florida, at the Barnes & Noble Bookstore.

My mom is 87 years old and one of her dreams has come true, her book is finally published. Her story about the trials of raising a son who had Cerebral Palsy (CP), *All His Fingers and Toes*, was written up today in the Naples Daily News, the News Press of Bonita Springs, and Naples Illustrated magazine will also be covering her story. I am so proud of my mother and her accomplishments. I am proud of how she dedicated her life to helping the handicapped.

The Barnes & Noble has a large table set up by the front door, and I brought my mother six long-stem roses which I set there. She is wearing a bright-orange blouse and cannot believe that this event is being held for her. She keeps looking at a large poster placed at the entrance. Greeting all entrants, it reads: "Event, join us for a signing: Rose Weiss, Author." People have already read about the book-signing party in the local Naples Daily News and have called in to reserve copies of my mom's book. Others are waiting in line to get my mother's autograph and speak to her. There is even a young man with Cerebral Palsy buying a book. All of the proceeds from one of the cash registers were donated to my brother's home, Woodhouse, in Dania, Florida.

My mother looks up at me and says, "Is this really happening?" I reply, "Yes, mom, it is. Your book is finally published."

Two decades earlier in 1980, part of my mother's book had been published in the Tropic Section of the Miami Herald. She and my brother were on the cover, under their picture the title of the article read: "All his Fingers and Toes, A story of what a mother's love can do." A long, twenty-year journey separated that article from the eventual publication of the book. My mother had been through countless trials trying to get her manuscript accepted by publishing houses. The prevailing feeling had been that although it was a touching story that had merit, and marketing reasons prohibited anyone from taking the project on.

After twenty years of failed attempts at getting her story published, my mother had given her crusade up. At this point my mother was in her eighties, and understandably exhausted. I thought that helping my mother get her book published would not be an impossible mission because of my prior writing experience.

After speaking with a friend at a wedding who had a contact with Health Communications, Inc the publishers of the Chicken Soup series of books, in Deerfield Beach, Florida, I gained a new incentive to further pursue this lifelong goal of my mothers. I worked with Health Communications, Inc. for a year trying to get to my mother's story published. In the end they turned down her story for marketing reasons as well. Health Communications said that I should still try to get the book published, that they loved the story and thought that it had value.

It wasn't until one night, at Barnes & Noble (which, ironically, my husband calls "The Library" because a lot of people sit in the store's comfortable chairs, reading the latest publications and books for free) that the process began to gather momentum. That night, I picked up a brochure about a company called iUniverse.com. My stepson checked into it and found that iUniverse was an on-line publishing company where people can send in a disk that contains a manuscript, edit it, design the cover, and for a modest price get their book published in about three months.

Prior to working with iUniverse, my only experience in publishing came from my years as an architecture graduate and interior designer. During that period of time, my own work had been published in local and national magazines and in books. Due to my limited experience in book editing, I asked my neighbor's son, Jonathan Spafford, a high school Junior, for help. He did the actual on-line editing, and when his work was done the book was ready for publication.

When Jonathan attended the book-signing party he found a receptive audience interested in hiring him to help with their editorial needs. What an accomplishment for a high school student two years away from graduation! Jonathan is now a film editor for a television show called "The Doctors" and has also been an assistant editor for many major motion pictures that have been released over the past several years. I have always considered myself good at detecting hidden talents in people. It was something that my mother had instilled in me when she taught me that the best help could often come from the least likely places. While I was talking to Jonathan at the party, a very polite, well-dressed man who worked at the bookstore overheard me telling him that he should sell his services. The man turned towards me and said, "Well, aren't you a tiger." In that instant, I knew that my father was also there in spirit because that was my father's pet name for my mother until his passing in 1973, just before my graduation from the University of Florida.

My mother never did care for fame; she merely wanted her story to be inspirational to other families that had children afflicted with CP. In this way, she felt, they would know that they were not alone. She wanted them to know, through her example, how to make their children's lives as normal as possible.

In a very real sense, it was her persistence that made my brother walk when most doctors said that it was an impossible dream.

My brother learned to write despite physical hardships as well. She never heeded the admonishments to keep him safe at home; rather she did her best to expose him to all that a normal life had to offer. She always knew that when you wanted something deep in your heart, you had to be persistent and never give up that dream. This is one of the greatest qualities that I inherited from her, a quality that I am very proud of to this day, a quality that has led me, sometimes through her urging, to excel in everything that I have done.

It was this same quality that guided her in her quest to help the handicapped. Over the years, she raised almost 600,000 dollars for the Sunland Training Center in Miami, the facility in which my brother lived for many years. My mother's desire to help was never solely directed towards my brother; instead it was extended to all the members of the place he lived as well. If my brother was taken out to eat, she paid for the whole group to join him. "You need to help them all" she always said, "It is the only proper thing to do." Her efforts over the years, among other things, allowed the center to install air-conditioning units in the housing facilities. The residents were so thankful to my mom because she made the lives of all the people there better during the long, hot, humid Florida summers. These were just some of the later fundraising efforts that had begun with the birth of my brother, almost sixty years prior.

It took my mother almost twelve years to get pregnant again and chance having a normal child. My brother was born with CP due to a doctor's error, which left him without oxygen during the first critical moments of his life. One can only wonder how scared she was when she found out that she was expecting me. Just as she taught me, though, you can accomplish anything, achieve any desire, if you work hard and never get disappointed—even in the face of failure. This book is her story as much as it is mine, and it is a story that needs to be heard.

CHAPTER 2
My Beginnings

My life started on October 7, 1950, at the old Mt. Sinai Hospital in Miami Beach, Florida. It was a miracle considering twelve years, one month, and one day earlier, my brother Elliott had been born at home in California, Pennsylvania, with Cerebral Palsy.

My mother made sure that I experienced everything that life had to offer. I played every sport imaginable, from ice-skating to basketball, and won prizes and accolades in many of the things in which I participated in grade school. I won second place in a "round the world" basketball competition. At summer camp I learned archery and riflery and won awards for both. I even won a first-place prize for my Easter egg design in the third grade. In high school I went on to win trophies for ballroom dancing, high-score awards in bowling, and second place in the Dade County Youth Fair for my linoleum-block print.

My mother said that I had always done well in school. In retrospect, I think that I was driven by the feeling that I had to compensate my parents for the things that they would never be able to get from my brother. To this end, I always strove to excel and eventually graduated with honors from Miami High in 1968. Initially, I went to University of Miami to be near my family, but eventually had to transfer to University of Florida to pursue my dream of becoming an interior designer. Before graduating in 1973, I was on the Dean's List several times and was a member of the School of Architecture's Gargoyle Honor Society.

After graduation, I got a job at the most prestigious architectural firm in Florida, Spillis Candela, located in Coral Gables, and began working on educational facilities. One of my first projects was the renovation of the cafeteria at the Sunland Training Center, the state institution where my brother Elliott lived. While with the firm, I worked under the same architect for eighteen years, a man who as a young boy had been flown from Cuba to the United States to be cured of Polio.

These relationships with people who had overcome adversity followed me through life and always had a positive effect on my own outlook. Little did I know, while working for this man I would eventually meet my future husband, Albert. In 1979 we purchased an old house in the historical Chinese Village district in Coral Gables. Although the house had fallen into disrepair we diligently worked to restore it to its original splendor. I won several awards for my efforts, and the house was featured in nationally recognized magazines and books.

I was once told by my best friend that I could never be normal with a brother like Elliot. I realized that this is not always a bad thing because my brother's handicap and my mother's resolution helped forge my own determination and consequently made me a better person.

Later in life Elliott was only home for holidays. His room became my mother's office, when he wasn't there. It was from this room that she conducted her fund-raising efforts for the handicapped. Notwithstanding her work in this area, she was always there for me, taking the time to talk to me about her experiences. Coupled with my own need to excel, these talks helped to make me an over-achiever and gave me the positive attitude that would follow me through life. It was this attitude that led me to play male-orientated sports, enter a male-dominated profession, and drove me back to school for my second degree, in architecture, while working full time as an interior designer.

To this day, my husband and friends often make jokes by saying that there is something that I cannot do. This only incites me to do it with more resolution and intensity than ever because in all my life I have never shied away from challenges and difficulties.

While cleaning out my mother's apartment after her sudden death from a fall in January, 2003, I found a black and white flowered suitcase. My mother had told me about the existence of a suitcase like this one, containing personal items from her life, but I had never actually seen it before. I picked it up and took it home with me, both afraid and curious of what I might find. For a couple of days, while I was mourning her death, I forgot about the suitcase. Instead, I thought of all of her life's achievements and disappointments. Finally, one night when I was by myself, I returned to the suitcase and unzipped it.

Like a whispered story, I began to discover Elliott through the eyes of my mother and my mother through mementos of him as I emptied the suitcase of their life together.

CHAPTER 3
Elliott's Birth

"He's not breathing."

These were the first words that my mother heard as my brother made his ominously silent entrance into the world. As she looked around see what was happening, she silently prayed that she had not heard correctly. It could not be her baby! She saw the doctor move rapidly and she held her breath as he put his mouth on the infant's lips, breathing quickly in and out in attempt to infuse life into the tiny body which was so deathly still. But then, suddenly, my baby brother began breathing rhythmically, properly, and she also took a deep breath, trying to calm down and convince herself that everything was all right.

Dr. Craft lifted the baby boy by his legs and spanked him lightly on the buttocks to get the customary first cry, but the baby remained silent. And then there was movement. A tiny leg jerked and extended to full length. She caught the new hope in nurse Sarah's eyes and she clung to this thought. Dr. Craft rose slightly again, and the tiny creature in his hands waved angry fists at him. But still he made no sound. No sound! Newborn babies cried. Even with her very limited experience, she knew this for a fact. Why wasn't her son crying? How could she tell her husband that their new son was not perfect?

It was early evening on September 8, 1938 and Elliott, her first-born, had arrived. He was bathed, dressed, and handed to her to be admired. She later told me that he looked so angelic, his face like a cherub, his eyes bright and alert. She could not detect anything about him that was not perfect in shape or form. He had all his fingers and toes. She knew for sure because she had examined each one and had counted them several times.

My father, Eddie, sat by the side of her bed and tenderly pulled back the receiving blanket to glimpse a better look at his son's face.

My mother said, "Eddie, he's so quiet. You don't think he's mute?"

"Rose, he's not mute." My father made little cooing noises at the child cradled in my mother's arms. "He'll cry soon enough... Just look at him, Rose. Have you ever seen a better looking baby?"

She knew that newborns take some time to get over the trauma of birth before they start to look cute, but she said that Elliott was an exception. From the blonde fuzz on the top of his head to the tiny toes on each foot, he seemed like a normal, healthy, perfect baby. He had a round face, good color, very few wrinkles, and his eyes were wide open. And each time she saw my beautiful baby brother, her heart reached out to him with love and kindness.

The first few times she tried to feed Elliott, she offered him the prepared formula Dr. Craft had prescribed, but much to her dismay, Elliott was unable to get his lips around the nipple, and when he tried, it kept falling from his mouth. In vain, she repeatedly tried to breast-feed. Tears formed in her eyes. She asked herself, "Why were my baby and I being punished?" They had done nothing wrong. She took all the vitamins regularly and ate the right foods during her pregnancy. She did not drink or smoke. So why were they being punished?

She asked Sarah, the nurse, to please bring an eyedropper and fill it with milk. To their joy, it worked! Part of the milk dribbled onto Elliott's chin, but he did retain some, at least enough to sustain him. This would be the first of many challenges and creative solutions that my family was about to encounter.

It was forty-eight hours before Elliott began to utter his first cry. Those early frantic wails filled our house like a joyous symphony. My mother said a deep prayer and reassured herself that now everything would be all right.

After Elliott's nap the next day, Sarah brought Elliott to my

11

mother to be nursed; however, she had a concerned look on her face. Elliott had a strange, brownish-yellow cast to the whites of his eyes and his flesh was not the beautiful pink it had been at birth. Sarah said it looked like jaundice. She maintained that Elliott's liver was not mature enough yet and that he needed more sunlight.

For nine months she had lived with her child growing inside her, and so her entire being was centered around her hopes and aspirations for this new life that she would give to the world. It is impossible for a mother to conceive anything but a perfect image, and when this image becomes reality it must conform, in every way, to the ideal you have established. Any inconsistency becomes enormous.

She should have faith in our doctor, she kept repeating in her mind. He told her that the baby was fine; that he was healthy and would grow up to be happy and tall and wonderful. Despite the doctor's optimistic words, she was still afraid.

The jaundice lasted for three weeks. During that time she experienced every doubt and fear a mother could conjure up. Perhaps it would have been easier to cope if he had possessed an abnormality that she could have seen or an illness that she could understand. Instead, her child had a quiet discontent that was shaped by her imagination into horrible life-threatening maladies. Everyone tried to help her. My father would sit by her bedside, holding her hand, and tell her what a wonderful child they had, but she could always hear the doubts in his voice. Sarah was steadfast in her determination that Elliott was normal, but she did not believe her either. A mother knows these things.

At the end of the week, Dr. Craft returned to check on my parents and brother. He examined the baby carefully, shining lights in his eyes, testing his reflexes, probing his skin with his fingertips. Dr. Craft was smiling when he came to my mother. He promised her that everything was going to be all right. He said, "I must admit that Elliott

12

is a little slow getting started, but I still believe that he is going to be a fine, healthy child. The respiration problem he had in the beginning is holding him back a little. But that is all."

How my mother wished that Dr. Craft was right! But, Elliott wasn't just a slow baby. There was something wrong and it became increasingly clear in the frequent trips she made to the doctor's office in the weeks that followed.

So many times she heard mothers declare that they wish their children would be more quiet or less of a bother to them, but she was praying for my child to make a fuss and to stop being such a "perfect baby." He slept constantly, and most of his waking hours were quiet ones. But he was also beautiful so she clung to her faint hopes that my worries were unfounded. Such a handsome infant could not possibly have anything seriously wrong with him.

My mother said that looking back, and even at the time, she wondered if things might have turned out differently for Elliott if he had been born in the hospital, but that was not always an option in the late 1930's, particularly in a town as small as California, PA. Most of my father's pharmacy business came from Dr. Craft, one of the busiest physicians in town, and so it wouldn't have been prudent to have another doctor deliver their child. My father insisted that Dr. Craft was a qualified physician, but my mother kept having terrible nagging doubts, and their child's lack of progress soon backed them up.

Elliott had weighed 7 pounds, 14 ounces at birth. Because they weren't feeding him from a bottle or the breast at first, Elliott gained weight slowly. When he tried to eat, he often gagged on the formula, which caused him to retain only a small portion of his food. She suspected that this was the heart of the problem. When Elliott was about a month old, they were elated when he finally learned to swallow his food, and in a short time, he grew 2-1/2 inches and gained 3 pounds. There was hope.

13

When Sarah's month with us came to an end, she took a position to care for another newborn. Now Elliott was solely in my mother's care. She tried to make him hold a rattle and play with his nursery toys, but he could not grasp them, nor did he show any interest in them. This made my parents more aware of a possible muscle handicap. It was then that my mother began to wonder if Elliott would ever sit, walk, or talk.

During the next few months, Elliott still showed no interest in his toys or rattles. My mother became more alarmed as he did not show the normal desires of babies. At night she would lie awake and worry, "What was his future going to be like? How could she help?"

On our long outings in the crisp air, she constantly showed Elliott the beautiful leaves and explained the different colors to him. They had one-way conversations, but she didn't care. He was all she had to talk to during these walks and she believed he heard her, despite his inability to respond. Their walks usually led us to see daddy at the drugstore where they would say hello to the customers.

Dressed in his white bunting suit, Elliott looked like a doll. But a closer look would reveal that he was tied into the carriage and propped up from behind with a pillow; otherwise, his body slumped over and his head flopped about uncontrollably. Even when carrying her baby around the house, she supported his little head by cupping it with the palm of her hand. Inwardly, she prayed Elliott would awaken one day soon and be perfectly normal. Instead, the days stretched into months and Elliott's problems became more evident.

The ritual circumcision, or bris, which is customarily performed on Jewish boys at the age of seven days old, was delayed because of Elliott's abnormality. But finally, at six weeks old, the doctor decided it should take place. With all of Elliott's feeding problems, he now had to be confronted with a surgical procedure. My mother was against doing it, but my father and other men in the family

14

insisted that the procedure was customary and that it had to be done.

It was a very emotional day. Their small apartment overflowed with family and friends. We selected my grandfather's brother, Emil, to be the godfather, so it was his privilege to hold Elliott during the circumcision. My father's mother took care of all the arrangements. She prepared the food and brought her housemaid to serve and clean up.

Elliott let out a loud cry when the foreskin was cut; however, a few moments later, with wine spattered on his lips, he quietly went to sleep and all was calm. When he fell asleep, my mother was bombarded with questions about his eating and sleeping habits and about what progress he was making. With each answer she became more and more disturbed. She wanted everyone to vanish quickly. She did not want more questions for which she had no answers, only doubts.

My mother didn't know what month a baby is first expected to hold a rattle or kick his feet or sleep through the night. She was a new mother. She had to learn from experience. She had not read any books about babies. My mother thought motherhood came naturally. She thought motherhood brought daily joy.

CHAPTER 4
Diagnosis and Move to Florida

When Elliott was about eight months old, my mother hired a professional photographer to take some portrait-style photographs. She was busy in the kitchen when she heard a sharp rapping on the front door. She found the photographer standing on the front porch, grinning broadly while he struggled to hold up an awkward collection of reflectors, lights, and tripods.

"Mrs. Weiss? Good morning! I'm from the studio."

"Yes, we've been expecting you," my mother said holding open the screen door. "Please come in."

The man started through the doorway, banged his Graflex on the frame, re-angled, and entered calmly on the second try. With cords dangling and tripods rattling loudly, he struggled into the living room and gratefully surrendered his burden onto the couch. Brushing his hands together with satisfaction, he looked around the room.

"There now. Where's our subject?"

"I'll get him. Would you like some coffee?"

"When I'm finished, thanks. It'll only take a minute."

My mother hesitated nervously and went into the nursery, lifting Elliott from his crib. She had already dressed him in his best outfit and he looked at her with anticipation as she carried him into the living room. The photographer came over, smiling, and inspected his newest client.

"Well, aren't you a good-looking fellow? Maybe we'll send your portrait off to Gerber so they can put you on their cereal boxes." He laughed at his own joke, a joke he probably made dozens of times per month. He tweaked Elliott's cheek, and then he was all business. "OK, Mrs. Weiss, we'll sit him on a table over here by the window, and I'll place the backdrop over here."

"Fine," my mother said hesitantly. "I'll get the blanket."

"Oh, we won't need that, ma'am. I've got all the props."

"You don't understand," she insisted, "I'll need the blanket to support him from behind. So you won't see my hands."

He looked at her strangely. "How old is your boy?"

"Eight months."

"Then he can hold his head up just fine. It'll be all right. We know what we're doing," he said, suddenly referring to himself in the plural tense. We've photographed a million kids just his age."

I've never understood why people retreat into the editorial "we" when they're trying to explain that they know more about something than you do? It's a habit I've noticed in crooked politicians and befuddled appliance repairmen. Before my mother could say another word, the photographer hustled off to set up the backdrop and the lights. She followed him, still persistent.

"I'm afraid you don't understand. Elliott's a slow child. He has difficulty doing things for himself." She realized as she said it that she'd never used the term "slow" before to refer to my brother.

"Sitting up comes naturally, Mrs. Weiss. He can do it fine on his own. No need to be overprotective. Just watch." The man put the backdrop in place, whisked Elliott from my mother's arms, and carried him to the waiting table.

"All right, captain, we want you to sit right here and smile for the little birdie," he commanded. He sat Elliott on the table and immediately, Elliott doubled over. "Come on, son. Sit up for me." There was a note of exasperation in the photographer's voice. "No time to fall asleep now. Sit up for the camera."

Elliott's head rolled uncontrollably.

"Come on, boy." The man's face was beginning to wrinkle with impatience. It was apparent that Elliott wasn't going to respond for him. He looked at my mother. "I suppose there is something wrong with your boy, Mrs. Weiss."

There was no longer any question. Elliott had smiled at three weeks and laughed at three months. He could drink from a cup, and by all outward appearances he was normal, yet he had no control over his body. He couldn't hold up his head or sit unaided. And at times when other babies would have started crying, Elliott was still as languid as a newborn. As the pictures were being taken, my mother propped Elliott up, holding him in place, her hands under his blanket, just as my father and her had done when taking amateur snapshots in the past.

My mother wasn't lacking from advice on ways to help Elliott. Everyone had a formula.

Later that month, my father's mother visited from Monessen, a nearby city where one of his brothers was living. Recently widowed, she was a short, imposing woman with the authority of having raised thirteen children of her own, as well as innumerable grandchildren. She carried the conviction of her Hungarian upbringing and an intense aura of command as she entered the house and settled into a living room chair.

"Bring me my grandson," she said, and my father rushed to bring forth Elliott and lay him in her arms. She bounced the child lightly against her breast for a moment, looking at him skeptically. Elliott's head rolled wildly in her arms.

"His muscles are too loose," she announced, as though it were something that had escaped our attention.

"We know, Mama," my father told her. "He's not coming along very fast."

"He needs starch," she proclaimed.

"Starch?" my mother asked, thinking that she meant Hungarian pasta or potatoes.

"Starch," she repeated. "Rose, you must bathe him in starch water. Potato starch. It will make him stiff like the collar of a new shirt. Do it often and he'll be well. I know. It's what we did in the Old Country."

At least my father's mother could suggest a cure, no matter how misdirected or confused. Dr. Craft was much less help. My mother could see that he was becoming increasingly uncomfortable with my regular visits to his office. His routine showed little variation. He would take Elliott's temperature, stretch his arms and legs, and peer into the baby's eyes. Always, at the end of the examination, he would shake his head and then tell my mother the same sort of nonsense: "He should start coming around now, Mrs. Weiss. He's a healthy baby. Just still a little slow."

The morning, after one of these examinations, my mother planned my next course of action. With breakfast on the table, she waited with anticipation while my father finished his shachrit, the morning prayers, in the bedroom. My mother formed my argument carefully while she waited, listening for the sound of his footsteps coming from the bedroom. He reached the doorway of the kitchen and stopped for a moment, suddenly clutching the door-frame and shaking his head.

"Eddie, what's wrong?" my mother asked.

He waved her off with his hand.

"It's nothing. I got up too quick and it made me a little dizzy." My father didn't look all right. His color was flushed.

"You're sure? Eddie, you don't look like you feel well. All we need is for you to get sick now," said my mother.

"I'm all right." He smiled reassuringly and came over to the breakfast table. My mother studied him carefully as he sat down and took the first sip of coffee, the color beginning to flow back into his cheeks.

19

"You didn't sleep well last night, either, Eddie," said my mother.

"My stomach was bothering me. Probably just a touch of the flu."

"It's been happening a lot lately."

"Please, Rose. It's nothing." From the tone in his voice she could tell that he didn't want to talk about it any further, but he knew she wasn't going to let him off that easily. He added, as an insincere concession, "If it gets any worse, I'll ask Dr. Craft about it."

"Dr. Craft is what I want to talk to you about," she said, deciding to go ahead with her original plan. She sat down across from my father at the table and said, "I don't think he's helping Elliott." My father began to spoon his cereal. He wasn't looking at her.

"He's delivered and raised a lot of healthy children, Rose."

"But he's not helping ours. I know he's a good friend, Eddie, and an important client of ours, but what if he's not good enough to help Elliott? What if he feels guilty about something that happened when the baby was born? Perhaps he gave me too much medication to induce labor, or he maybe he shouldn't have tried so hard to get Elliott to breathe at first. Couldn't he have known that there might be damage later on?"

My father looked at my mother sharply. "Rose, that's a terrible thing to say. Wilson's a good man and a very well-respected doctor."

"I know, Eddie, I know," she said." The tears she didn't want forced their way into her eyes. "I know he's a good man, Eddie, but he just hasn't been good enough. I want someone else to look at our son before it's too late."

My father went back to his cereal, chasing it around the bowl with his spoon, but he wasn't eating. Finally, he nodded. "Maybe a second opinion won't hurt, so long as you don't see another doctor here in town. Dr. Craft doesn't need to know about our private business."

"Let's take him to Pittsburgh. There are good doctors there."

"Absolutely," my father said. "I'll make some calls and see if I can't get us the name of a good pediatrician in the city."

"Let's do it, Eddie, right away, while we can still help our son."

My father came up with a lot of names in the weeks that followed, but most of them were pediatricians with small office practices, and in their own way they were as knowledgeable and helpful as Dr. Craft. They would go in for an examination, then sit in an endless series of wood-paneled offices while kindly doctors reclined in their leather executive chairs or perched on the corner of immense oak desks to give their verdicts. Each doctor had a different opinion: muscular problems, malnutrition, nervous ailments, bone diseases. None of these ideas rang true, but my parents tried each of their suggestions for treatment: large doses of vitamins, a sun lamp, rigid diets, and countless other remedies. They all had the same effect, or lack thereof.

At first, my father was tolerant of the interminable series of tests and examinations. Although he didn't speak much, he confessed that Elliott needed more help. He would often sit by his son's crib watching him, and he would say, "I just don't understand how the Lord could do this to such a beautiful child." In this matter, my parents agreed wholeheartedly.

My mother didn't realize how much the stress of the situation was troubling my father until one night at supper when he confessed that he had been in to see Dr. Craft for his own problems. He produced a small brown bottle and popped a white lozenge into his mouth as he began eating.

"What's that, Eddie?" my mother asked. Always the pharmacist, he explained it to my mother with a twenty-syllable

21

technical name.

"No, really," she insisted, "what is it?"

"A tranquilizer," he said, shuffling his food around on his plate moodily. "Wilson gave it to me for my stomach problem and the dizzy spells."

"What's wrong, Eddie?" my mother asked urgently.

"Nothing organic, Rose. Don't worry yourself. It's only stress."

"Is something wrong at work?"

"Oh, just the usual." He nodded toward the high chair where Elliott had been strapped into place, supported by a pillow, while they ate. "I just worry about him too much, I guess. Dr. Craft wants me to relax a little more."

My father turned to his food again, making it clear that this was all that we were going to discuss about the matter. Elliott gurgled beside him, his bright eyes staring at his father.

My mother had not realized the reassurances that she had demanded from my father, or that she had pressured him so greatly when he put on his strong, comforting facade. In general, their home life had been good over the last year. The house was frequently filled with friends and relatives who seemed to overlook Elliott's misfortunes as they showered their affection upon him. My parents even took turns baby-sitting so that each of us could enjoy an occasional night out. Prior to this, my father had never let on that their son's affliction was eating away at him. But that night, my mother came to realize that Elliott's problems were a constant emotional burden to him, just as they were for her.

Elliott and my mother visited the store every day, and it seemed to take some of the pressure off of my father. He would lift Elliott out of the carriage and carry him down the aisles of bright packages and exotic-looking bottles. My mother stood by the counter, watching her

22

son enjoy the daily inventory with his father.

"Well, what do you think of this dusty old drugstore, boy? Do you like all the pretty bottles?" Elliott cooed contentedly. "See that? Mom puts that stuff on her fingernails." My brother grabbed for the bottle. "No, no, sorry, not for you. Look over here. See that? Jellybeans. Pretty Soon you can have one. What do you think of that? Which one would you like?"

The front door jangled as a customer wandered into the store. My father looked up at him, smiling, still holding Elliott.

"Good morning, sir. Can I help you?"

"Well, I'll be," the man said, only half joking. "This *is* a real baby."

"Yes," my father said quietly. "He's my son."

"I never would have known. He stays so beautiful and still. Just passing by and looking through the window, I would have thought it was a little doll you were holding." The man tickled Elliott under the chin and wandered off down an aisle. My mother could see the resignation wash over my father's face. Silently, he handed Elliott back to my mother and went back behind the pharmacy counter. The stress was still there, and the lack of knowing anything conclusive weighed heavily on both of them. But if none of the doctors understood, what could they do? Before long it, they knew that it would be impossible to hide the fact that Elliott was handicapped.

It was a bitter word, but she was beginning to use it more and more often in her mind. There was something less than normal about my brother. When a person is afflicted, one must first learn the name of the malady that possesses him in order to fight it. They felt that way with Elliott, and if they could only put a label on the problem, then maybe they would be able to defeat it. Instead, they had a beautiful child who wasn't progressing, who remained flaccid, but usually smiled in their arms.

23

She strapped Elliott into the carriage and was ready to head out when a regular customer entered the store. It was a man wearing a herringbone overcoat over a three-piece suit. He pushed a teenage boy before him in a large wicker carriage. The boy's head rolled unnaturally to the side, like Elliott's, and his hands and legs were twisted at odd angles. The man smiled sheepishly at her and directed his son over to the ice cream counter. My mother stood rooted to the spot, watching as he ordered a dish of vanilla ice cream and then patiently spooned it into his son's mouth, wiping away the drool that inevitably spilled out. Feeling weak, she turned back to my father and saw he had been watching as well. Her eye caught his and he turned away, retreating to the back of the store.

Our son will never be like that, or have to be fed by someone, she told herself, looking down at Elliott in the stroller. But first they had to find out what was wrong and deal with it. There just wasn't any other way.

A few weeks later my mother bought a new stroller with a metal plate on the bottom where a child could rest his feet, but Elliott was already a little big for it, so she removed the plate and left him sitting in the stroller in the living room. The first time she put him into it, he was still for a moment, and then he stretched his foot out tentatively to touch the floor. His tiny shoe pressed against the rug as if testing it, and then surprisingly, he shoved. The stroller moved a few inches backward. Elliott giggled and looked around. He stretched his foot out again and shoved again. The stroller rolled slowly toward the couch and bounced to a stop.

Elliott was propped up with a pillow, but he could look around. His brow wrinkled in concentration and he shoved again, this time moving the stroller at a slight angle from the couch.
The back door opened and my father came in, exhausted from a long day at the store. He saw my mother standing transfixed in the living

room entrance and came over curiously to see what was going on.

"He's moving, Eddie," my mother told him. "Elliott's moving on his own."

Elliott grunted and shoved again, and the stroller went forward this time. He trundled over to the coffee table and began diligently exploring. My parents looked at one another in amazement.

Yes. For the first time, Elliott was moving about on his own. It was a start.

Elliott pushed his stroller around the corner of one of the drugstore aisles, saw what he was looking for, and homed in on it. Sticking his tongue out of the corner of his mouth with determination, he navigated between the magazine racks and shampoo bottles to the large barrel of jellybeans at the candy counter. As he reached the candy counter, he came to a bumping stop and then stretched over the top to scoop out a handful of jellybeans. Oblivious to everything happening around him, he awkwardly drew in his prize, holding it in his lap while he picked out the black beans first, chewing them with obvious delight.

"That shows he can pick out colors and demonstrate a preference," my father told my mother from their vantage point by the pharmacy counter. "And he's getting around better. Maybe he'll be normal after all."

"He still needs help, Eddie," my mother insisted. "Aunt Tillie and Uncle Julius want me to go see a doctor they know in Miami. He's an orthopedist. Tillie and Julius wouldn't have recommended him if they didn't think he might be able to help. They love Elliott very much."

"Florida is a long way," my father replied doubtfully. "I don't know if I want you going so far away."

"It's for Elliott's sake, Eddie. If there's a way to help him, we have to try it."

25

"Are you sure you're not just sick of the Pennsylvania winter?"

"The winters here are difficult," my mother conceded, "but it's Elliott that I'm concerned about, Eddie. He's so sickly . . . I think Miami will be good for him."

My father's fingertips drummed on the counter as he thought about it.

"Well, maybe. We've tried everything else. And you need a vacation. As long as you don't get in the habit."

As they continued to struggle with Elliott's mysterious deformities, events were taking an ominous turn in the rest of the world. President Roosevelt had gone against the nationwide isolationist sentiments to ask Congress to provide a Lend-Lease program to aid the Allies, and at the same time he submitted a mammoth $17.5 billion budget to Congress that included $11 billion for defense. It seemed as though the government knew it would be drawn into war. In response, many influential senators and business leaders had joined together to establish the America First Committee in an attempt to keep us out of the war, although it meant abandoning our nation's friends overseas and, in particular, the millions of Jews we knew Hitler was persecuting in the occupied countries.

The threat of war was driving prices upward rapidly, making it doubly hard to meet their payments for Elliott's tuition. My father had difficulty stocking many of the items that were normally carried in the store, from chocolate to important medicines.

Despite the adversity, the country seemed bursting with hope and creativity. Production was picking up, partly due to the large defense expenditures, and the Depression was, at last, truly over. Americans were responding with fantastic works, from the stone heads of Mount Rushmore, to the great literary works that were beginning to emerge. F. Scott Fitzgerald had died the previous December, leaving behind *The Last Tycoon,* which was just being published posthumously, sharing the shelf with *What Makes Sammy Run?* and *The Keys to the Kingdom*—all reflecting new faith in the economy or the magnitude of power at the top. *Citizen Kane*, *The Maltese Falcon*, and *Sergeant York* were showing at the movies, and the radio was playing "Chattanooga Choo-Choo," "The Boogie-Woogie Bugle Boy," and "The Jersey Bounce." It was a bold, bright time before the gathering darkness.

It was a cold, drizzly day when my mother and Elliott boarded the train in Pittsburgh. Soldiers and sun-bound tourists filled the passenger cars and the brilliant domed observatories. Elliott chortled with excitement as the train pulled from the station and the panorama outside the windows began to unfold. As they passed houses, farms, and small villages, she told Elliott stories about them as he watched in wide-eyed amazement.

"Do you see that farm? It's Old MacDonald's farm. See his horses? Do you know what kind of sound those cows make? Moo-oo."

Elliott laughed happily and bounced on my mother's knee, she supported him from behind by her carefully placed hand. Across the aisle, fellow travelers smiled warmly at him. Despite his excitement, the gentle rocking of the train soon lulled him to sleep, and by the time the warm morning light streamed through the windows, they were in Florida. An entirely new vista of palm trees and palmetto shrub stretched around them. Cattle grazed on open plains, and the sky was clearer and brighter than it ever seemed in Pennsylvania.

As they stepped out into the warm, invigorating air at the train station in Miami, Tillie and Julius were there to meet them. They grabbed Elliott from my mother and squeezed him with genuine affection, and he burbled back a happy sound in response, his arms and legs flailing in a worm-like, disjointed manner.

"It's good to see you, little one," Julius told Elliott. "We've got

27

a man here who is going to make you all better. What do you think of that?"

His eyes sparkled with confidence as he said it, and Tillie patted my mother's hand comfortingly. She tried to share their enthusiasm, but as always the doubt and apprehension plagued her.

They unwound for a few days before making their appointment with Dr. Kaiser. He gave Elliott one of the most thorough examinations the boy had ever had, while my mother hung back, trying to keep out of the way. Finally, they were led into his office and offered a chair.

"Please sit down, Mrs. Weiss. I think you were wise to bring Elliott down to see us."

"Can you help him?" my mother asked.

"I'm afraid it's impossible to tell you anything definite. Any sort of prognosis we could make for your son would be based largely on guesswork. The boy's determination will ultimately decide how much he will be able to accomplish, particularly in the area of expressive language."

She felt her hopes sinking yet again, but at least Dr. Kaiser hadn't mentioned a physical disability. It would be all right, somehow, even if he couldn't talk, if he could only get about by himself. He was doing so well with the stroller...

"What about walking, doctor?"

"There again, it's difficult to say. Certainly physical therapy would help and it should be started as soon as possible. There's an excellent man down here I want to refer to you. His name is Dayton, O.W. Dayton, and he is extremely dedicated. If anyone can see to it that Elliott walks on his own, Dr. Dayton should be able to help."

Once Dr. Dayton had examined Elliott, my mother asked, "But what's the problem, doctor? Why can't he walk? What's holding him back?"

28

Dr. Dayton began to study his notes with a sudden interest. "I can't really say for sure. It's a difficult case, and the cause doesn't really matter. What we have to do now is find a way to make him better."

Dayton's advice turned out to be the first positive suggestion anyone had given my mother, and despite the cost, they enrolled Elliott in a therapy program five days a week. He worked with Elliott slowly, placing him on the matted floor and drawing one leg forward, then an arm, then another leg, then the other arm, always offering words of encouragement.

"There you go, Elliott. You can do it. Just a little more. One leg at a time. That's better."

And Elliott did it. As my mother watched, he put out one hesitant arm on his own, then followed with his leg, gradually hoisting his tiny body behind him. He was crawling.

Within a month, with daily encouragement from the dedicated therapist, Elliott learned to crawl for himself. My mother could see his face brighten with the feeling of power this gave him. He began crawling everywhere, investigating every room of Tillie and Julius' house. Every accessible drawer was yanked open, its contents spilled out and meticulously inspected. Rooms began to look as though they had been turned sideways, with every unsecured item swept to the carpet and scattered. It was wonderful.

Elliott learned to take Uncle Julius by the hand and every morning he lead him to the closet in their room. A low rod had been attached underneath all of Elliott's apparel. Elliott would point out what he wanted to wear that day and Julius would help him get dressed.

The therapy also awakened other areas of activity in Elliott. He began making specific sounds that were not yet words, but which had definite meanings—for food, for the bathroom, for play, to go outside. Julius and Tillie were constantly patient and understanding, and they were always there to cater to the needs of my brother.

Florida was different in those days. There was no annual migration of snowbirds coming to roost on the undeveloped beaches, and there had been, as yet, no mass exodus from Cuba. Instead, pristine Art Deco buildings mingled with red-tiled Mediterranean homes in a world of towering banyans, fruit-laden mango trees, and healthy palms. The pace was slow and intoxicating. They would sit in the yard on a tropical night in mid-winter, and it was hard for my mother to feel burdened with Elliott's problems. There was much love here, and my brother was making progress.

"We'd like you to leave Elliott here," Julius said to my mother one night.

"What?" The comment startled her and she looked up into his serious face. Tillie was sitting close to him, leaning forward in eager anticipation. It was obvious that they had been discussing this for quite some time, but my mother couldn't understand why.

"We want you to leave Elliott here with us. He's obviously making progress and..."

"Oh, Julius, thank you, but I couldn't leave him. And I do have to be getting back to Eddie soon. Who knows how long Elliott will need therapy?"

"It doesn't matter how long." Tillie spoke now, unable to contain herself any longer. "If he lives with us he will always be near his therapist, and here he can enjoy the sunshine all year. You see how he likes it. Rose, we can't have a boy of our own. If you let us, we can adopt him and really help him. You've got plenty of time for other children at your age. You could go home and have another."

My mother was startled. She sat back in her chair, uncertain how to reply. No one was going to take her son from her, no matter what his problem was.

30

Still, she could see the hope in their eyes. Tillie and Julius had been like parents to her, and she knew that the only shadow in Tillie's bright, good-natured world was the fact that she would always be childless. Tillie sat in her chair, small, plump and earnest, and it was hard not to sympathize with her. Julius would be a good father as well. He was often mistaken for Barry Goldwater and had the same conservative, well-humored nature. He patted his wife's hand softly and tried to put things into more rational terms.

"It's for your sake as much as Elliott's," he said quietly. "Give us a chance, Rose. We could make such a good home for the boy. You've seen how we've helped so far."

My mother stood up, confused and embarrassed by their gesture. "I think I had better go inside now. It's getting late." She tried to start for the door, but she knew she couldn't leave the matter open. "I appreciate the offer, I really do. But Elliott's *my* son. He's my only child. We've come so far together. You must understand." She left them sitting on the porch and hurried inside.

The next morning my mother remained in her room longer than usual. Elliott was crawling about on the floor, repeatedly going over to the door and trying to open it. He was confused about being shut in and kept looking at my mother questioningly, but she had no idea how she going to face Tillie and Julius again. She had explained her reasons, but knew it had taken tremendous courage for them to even ask her; and she hated to disappoint them after all they had done for Elliot. Finally, she composed herself, opened the door, and followed Elliott as he scampered toward the kitchen.

Things never go as you expect. She turned the corner to the kitchen table, and much to her surprise, my father was standing there with a cup of coffee in his hand.

"Surprise!" he said, beaming.

Elliott held back a moment, confused, and then sped over to his

31

father. My father laughed with delight and scooped his son into the air, grinning enthusiastically while Tillie and Julius looked on from the other side of the room.

"Look at you, Elliott! Crawling," my son is growing up."

My mother could hold back no longer. She rushed around the corner of the table and squeezed both of her men together.

"When did you get here, Eddie?" my mother asked.

"I arrived about twenty minutes ago," he said, letting Elliott slip down to the floor and go scooting away for his morning hug from Aunt Tillie. My father leaned over and kissed my mother on the lips.

"I missed you, Rose," he said softly.

"I missed you too, Eddie, but what are you doing here?"

"I drove down with a friend so we could spend a few days together before going home." He squeezed my mother. "We have to celebrate Elliott's progress."

From the safety of arms, I my father's arms, my mother watched the disappointment wash over Tillie's and Julius' faces. But it didn't matter. My mother had a family and she was determined to keep it together. That was her priority.

My mother and Elliott spent the next day introducing my father to the sights of Miami. Elliott, in particular, enjoyed the beach and a last chance to splash in the tepid ocean waters.   However, despite its growing reputation as an elite resort, Miami Beach still lacked most of the commercialism and tourist attractions that crowd it today. Fortunately, they were able to get away alone and enjoy each other in a momentarily perfect world.

On their last night, they celebrated with a special dinner with Tillie and Julius. When everyone had finished eating, Tillie and my mother retired to the kitchen with the dishes. She knew exactly what was on Tillie's mind.

"You haven't reconsidered, have you, Rose?"

"Tillie, I'm sorry, but I can't leave Elliott behind."

"Please remember that we asked because you live up north, Rose. Your uncle and I want him very much. If you can't get anyone to help the boy any more, we'd like to adopt him legally if we could, but we don't mean to suggest that he shouldn't be with his mother." She stopped washing the dishes for a moment, looking like she was about to cry. "You're always welcome here," she said. "All three of you."

"I appreciate it, Tillie. Really. But Elliott needs us and we can help him now. He's getting better."

A gale of laughter burst through from the other room. Tillie and my mother rushed to the doorway to see what was going on. Elliott was kneeling on the bathroom threshold, triumphantly clutching one end of a roll of toilet tissue. The rest of the roll left a labyrinth trail behind him, snaking in and out of the bathtub, around the sink, into the hall, and up and down the hall walls. Elliott's eyes were wide open with pride at his accomplishment.

And my mother was proud of him, too!

By the fall of 1940, Elliott was two years old and was still unable to stand erect, talk, or coordinate his leg muscles. He continued to have difficulty grasping and holding things, and was squirming and twisting as much as ever. My mother begged my father to let her see another doctor, the chief pediatrician at the Children's Hospital in Pittsburgh. After a lengthy discussion, he agreed.

They waited in the doctor's office while he examined Elliott. Then, while a nurse kept Elliott busy, the doctor came in and settled in his chair. They'd been through this routine with other doctors, but this time, the result was a bit clearer.

"Well, Mr. and Mrs. Weiss, I'll get right down to business," he said. "We know what's wrong with your child."

My mother felt her heart lurch and leaned forward in her chair.

"I'm afraid that Elliott is a spastic," the doctor told us. "It's a condition that results from brain damage early in life. The affliction manifests itself in a number of different ways, depending on the part of the brain that's been damaged."

"Damaged . . . but how?"

"Probably from the lack of oxygen for the first few moments when he was born. That's a terribly critical moment."

"But how can you be certain so quickly?" My mother's remaining hopes that Elliott would prove to be normal after all were rudely disappearing from sight.

"We're as certain as we can be. Mrs. Weiss, I've been with the Children's Hospital for quite a number of years now. We see a lot of things that the normal general practitioner in a small town never encounters. We've had children just like Elliott brought to us for diagnosis when other doctors have failed to identify the problem, through no fault of their own. We are a highly-acclaimed teaching hospital. We have little doubt as to the nature of the affliction or to its cause. I'm sorry."

My father gave my mother a warning look, certain that she was about to burst into tears, but she was too stunned. She could only sit there, wringing her hands and listening to the doctor.

"What does this mean exactly?" My father asked him.

"Well, there are a number of characteristics of a spastic child. Sometimes their heads wiggle helplessly, sometimes they're rigid, and sometimes they're overly mobile. Again, it depends on the nature of the damage to the brain."

"But will Elliott get well?" My mother asked.

"He'll always have a physical handicap to overcome, Mrs. Weiss. Damage to the brain doesn't go away. But I can venture a guess that he *will* be able to talk some day. However, most of these children don't develop the coordination to walk on their own."

"But what can my husband and I do to help him get better? There has to be something."

"You can take him home and feed him well. Try to keep him warm and comfortable and happy, Mrs. Weiss. And thank God for the blessings you *do* have."

"But what about school?"

The doctor's eyebrows arched and an edge of impatience crept into his voice. "School? No school would accept him, Mrs. Weiss. Even an institution is going to have too much difficulty caring for him properly. My best advice is for you to keep on as you've been doing."

"It's not right," my mother said to my father using a handkerchief to mop away the inevitable tears as they drove away from Pittsburgh. She held Elliott tightly in her lap, finally letting her anguish out.

"It's not right. Elliott has as much right to enjoy this world as anybody else. There has to be a way to save him from this kind of life."

"Rose," My father said carefully, "you've got to accept what the doctor told us. Together we have to care for Elliott the best way we can, but we can't build up our hopes too much. Just take things as they come and the Lord will give us the strength to do what we have to for Elliott. The Lord has a reason for making him this way, even if we can't see it right now. We just have to do the best we can."

The words were easy, but how does a mother come to terms with the fact that there is something definitely and permanently wrong with her son? She would now have to face that fact, Lord's will or not.

First, you try to place the blame on someone else. Many excuses came to mind. Dr. Craft must have given me too much medication at Elliott's birth or during the pregnancy itself. The prescriptions from the other doctors had harmed Elliott in some way. She had not been given proper consultations by her friends and parents

35

during her pregnancy, and something they had told her to do resulted in this thing that had happened to her boy. She wondered if the flu she had during the third month of pregnancy could have been a factor. She wondered lots of things, some more logical than others.

When none of these rationalizations worked, she blamed herself. Perhaps she had not eaten properly, or maybe the walks she had taken while she was pregnant had done him some harm. Could climbing the stairs day after day to their second floor apartment have caused him harm?

She went through the physical disabilities, then turned to the spiritual ones. You can really damn yourself with these thoughts. My mother thought perhaps it was punishment for not keeping strictly to her religion, for not being as devout as my father had been. Perhaps they had married too young, when we were untested, and God thought we needed an obstacle to overcome together. Perhaps she had not been good enough to my father and this challenge was meant to bring them closer together.

Her positive thoughts turned blacker after that. My mother thought "Perhaps there's no God at all, or perhaps there is a God but He's vengeful. Maybe there was some evil in me that was expressing itself through my child."

My father's faith was an encouragement to my mother. Perhaps it was because he was always so quiet, but he seemed so strong in his faith. He was thirty-three now and my mother felt protected by his maturity. If he said that this was the Lord's doing and that things would work out, then she had to cling to that thought.

In Judaism, there are many stories about dealing with adversity, stories that teach you to laugh at your misfortunes because things could always be far worse. One tale about a man in Poland who went to a *shadchen*, a professional matchmaker comes to mind. The matchmaker introduced him to a beautiful girl and he took her for a stroll through the park in Gdansk. After taking the girl home, he turned quickly to the shadchen and said, "This girl is beautiful, Mrs. Hinkel, but she has a terrible limp."

"Only when she walks," Mrs. Hinkel replied.

"That's how I should think of Elliott," she told herself. He's so beautiful, such a perfect baby. He snuggled close in her arms as the car climbed the hills out of Pittsburgh, and no one could have told by looking at him that there was anything wrong.

There's another story about Mrs. Hinkel. Another suitor returned to her one evening, livid, while his "date" sat just outside the door in their carriage. "You've swindled me," he hissed at her. "Never have I seen a creature as ugly as this one you've sent me out with. She's old, she's ugly as an old horse, she lisps, and she squints like a mole."

"There's no need to whisper," Mrs. Hinkel said. "She's deaf, too."

There was always that uneasiness, the chance that Elliott's disease would lead to further complications, or that there was something else wrong that they had not recognized yet.

Brain damage sounded so terrible, so final, so permanent. But people came back from strokes and learned to walk again. Wasn't a stroke a form of brain damage? People were injured in car accidents, or shot in the head in the war, and they survived and regained their faculties. Why should this disability with their son be so final? Why couldn't they find some way to overcome it?

She was in denial again, back where she had been long before the trip to Pittsburgh. At long last, here was a doctor who had experience with hundreds of these cases, yet he was telling her to go home and keep Elliott warm and comfortable and to expect no more progress for the rest of his life.

But how can you tell someone to live without hope? She

37

wouldn't have had the heart. She couldn't do it. And with that, the quest that would shape the rest of her life was well underway.

Even today, the medical facts seem inhuman and cruel in their analytical finality. Cerebral palsy strikes as the result of an injury to the brain at birth or shortly afterward. The disability has three major forms, depending on the location of the injury. What follows is what the doctor in Pittsburgh had tried to explain, facts which she could not comprehend in the midst of the terrible verdict:

The largest part of the brain is the cerebral cortex, the convoluted grayish tissue most of us think of when we speak of the brain. It is divided into four lobes of varying sizes: the frontal lobe, the parietal lobe, the temporal lobe, and the occipital lobe. The active nerve cells of the cortex, about eight billion of them, organize all the information that is fed into the brain from our various senses. If the injury occurs in this area of the brain, the result is the "spastic" form of cerebral palsy.

A much smaller section of the brain, located under the cortex, is the cerebellum. The brain centers its control of coordination and balance in the cerebellum. An injury to this section of the brain is called ataxia.

The third type of this disability strikes the brain stem or basal ganglia. It is called athetoid palsy. In most cases, the disability combines all three types of damage.

For a long time people with the disability were called "spastics" as a blanket reference, although the term, with all its cruel connotations, actually referred to only one form of the affliction. It has also been called Little's Disease, among many other much crueler names in the vernacular.

In spastic palsy, the victim's limbs move as a solid piece, making movement rigid and unnatural. If the victim ever learns to walk, he develops a scissors gait that makes the legs cross with every

38

step. Speech is difficult and the mouth drools almost constantly, a side effect that causes most people to automatically assume the victim of the disease is mentally impaired.

In contrast to this rigidity, in athetosis the victim has mobile spasms with involuntary, slow wiggling movements. When he tries to move, he has a writhing motion and his face contorts into weird grimaces, again leading people to believe that he is incapable of normal intelligence. Athetosis can also manifest itself in another form, chorea, an involuntary and irregular jerkiness of motion, which forces its victim to use a hopping gait.

Finally, there is ataxia. In many ways it is the worst of all the variations of cerebral palsy. This was Elliott's problem. Ataxia is a lack of balanced action between opposing muscle groups, with a consequent clumsiness of movement. The person with ataxia suffers from slurred speech, tremors, and a rolling or staggering gait like that of a drunken person. Muscles tend to be more flaccid than rigid. When the ataxic person tries to pick up something, he brings his arm down in a swoop—the classic description is "like an eagle on a rabbit." There is a disordered sense of position. The ataxic person is not always certain where his arms and legs are, or what they are doing. His mind is a parent to his limbs, which behave like a quartet of unruly children.

Each of the descriptions of the condition mentions what it is like for a person who is mobile—how the condition affects someone who is otherwise normal. My mother grasped that notion and then she remembered something else. Approximately a year earlier there had been an article in *Reader's Digest* about a doctor in Florida with cerebral palsy who spoke about his own struggle to overcome the malady, and how he subsequently established a residential school to treat the disability. Although she had not applied the story to Elliott's case when she first read the article, nor to the particular name of the demon that possessed Elliott, she later realized that the doctor was writing about the same condition that plagued Elliott. Now she knew the name of Elliott's condition, and she hoped that would help them to fight back.

When they arrived home, Elliott was asleep. While my father carried him upstairs, my mother went to the bookshelf to search through the back issues of my magazines for the article in *Reader's Digest*. She found the story quickly and reread it while my father was tucking Elliott into bed. He came out in a few minutes, stretched his arms to fight away the knots from the long drive, and sat down in his favorite chair.

"Rose, I'm sorry that it had to end like this, but I guess it's best to know just where we stand with this thing. We can still make Elliott a good home and be as much a family as possible, but now we know there's not much else for us beyond that."

"Eddie, I want to go to Florida again." My mother said.

He tilted his head to the side, clearly surprised at the conversation's new direction.

"Florida? I don't know if we can really afford another trip to see Tillie and Julius right now, Rose. I know they were good to you and Elliott and all but..."

"Eddie, there's another doctor."

There was a long moment of silence as my father stared at my mother, and she felt her resolve coming away at the edges. But she held on, and when my father didn't respond immediately, she plunged ahead.

"His name is Dr. Earl R. Carlson, and he's got the same things wrong with him that are wrong with Elliott. He couldn't control his muscles either. He couldn't speak. He was spastic-- just like Elliott-- and he beat it. He still struggles with his walking and with his speech, but now he's got a clinic in Florida and he's teaching other children."

"Rose, you heard what the doctor said today."

"Yes, but he never had to face the problem himself. Here's a man, just like Elliott, who says that with intensive training, concentration, and therapy, this thing can be beaten. The doctor beat this thing and now his patients are doing it. Eddie, this means there is hope as long as we act while Elliott's young enough to learn."

My father lowered his head, weighing the alternatives.

"I don't know, Rose. You have to think about this too. I don't know if I want you away from me that long. On the other hand, if you look into this school and you're convinced it looks like it might be good for Elliott, then I can't say no to you."

My mother wrote to Dr. Carlson, explaining in detail the diagnosis from Children's Hospital and their own observations of their son. As she wrote, the hopes built up inside her again.

But what if this man couldn't help Elliott either? What if he wouldn't see him? What if he wouldn't accept him into his program? What if it was more than we could afford? There was no one else to turn to, no one else who understood.

In spite of himself, my mother could see that my father was building up his expectations as well. He had read Dr. Carlson's article along with excerpts from his life story, *Born That Way*, which has become the classic text on the development cerebral palsy victims. Dr. Carlson had overcome severe physical handicaps to become a pediatrician so that he could treat others, who, like himself, were "born that way." That was Dr. Carlson's expression for children born with cerebral palsy, and he used that expression for the title of his own life story, *Born That Way*.

Dr. Carlson's book tells about his personal struggle for physical strength and emotional maturity in his attempt to make a place for himself in the world. Not surprisingly, my parents saw much promise in Dr. Carlson's words. When my mother told my father about her fears he would say, "We'll worry when the time comes, Rose. Don't borrow trouble right now. If Dr. Carlson can't take Elliott, maybe there will still be a way. Maybe we don't have to abandon all hope after all."

My parents were hoping again.

Chapter 5
Education or Lack Thereof

After two weeks that passed like years, my parents finally received a letter inviting them to bring Elliott to Pompano Beach, Florida for an examination by Dr. Carlson. By this time, Elliott, who was now almost four years old, had stopped improving at home. His awkward crawl remained the same and he still couldn't balance himself well enough to stand up. Walking, of course, was impossible for him.

As for his speech, Elliott was trying to learn new words, although his only recognizable words were "ma-ma" and "da-da." My mother spent every spare moment trying to expand his tiny vocabulary, pointing out things around him, patiently reciting their names and then searching for a coherent reply. "Ta-ble," "win-dow," "pup-py." Elliott seemed interested, staring at the place where she pointed and listening carefully at the name she gave the object. When it was something he liked, he would show obvious delight. And he was equally definite in things that he disliked. The words, however, were beyond his power. Awkward bodily gestures and contorted facial expressions continued to be his primary means of communication.

The Carlson School at Pompano Beach housed about 60 residents, ranging in age from 3 years old to adult, most of them quite severely handicapped. The majority of the residents came from wealthy homes. In the economy of 1940, the $160 monthly tuition was, as you can imagine, a tremendous sum for my parents to pay, but they were ready to sacrifice whatever was necessary to give their son the chance in life he deserved.

Dr. Carlson explained that many children made excellent progress within a year's time at his school, progress which enabled many of them to return to a relatively "normal" life. He conceded too, that some would remain with him for years. Admittedly, she was cautious, but what choices did they have?

As for Dr. Earl Carlson himself, his mother had saved him. She died when he was only 20, but during the years she was with him she refused to give up hope. When he fought her, she fought him harder. When he wanted to give up, she persevered. When he fell, she picked him up; when he was weak, she was strong. She made him walk and talk and learn, and in the end she made him more than a man—she made him great. My parents felt they could do no less for their son.

Years earlier, Dr. Carlson had fallen ill, and had called in a German nurse to take care of him. She had been gentle, patient, and loving. Before long, he regained his strength, married her, and together they founded a school for brain-damaged children on Long Island. Over the years it expanded from the nursery school level through high school, and then they opened a second facility in Florida. Now the residents of the school alternated between the facilities, spending the warm summers on the beaches of Long Island and the winters in the healthy Florida sun.

As my mother sat patiently, waiting through another interminable examination for Dr. Carlson's decision, she watched him work and drew strength from his own victory over the disease. He was a slightly built man with intense eyes and sallow features. Only the awkward position of his hands and the rolling manner in which he walked gave a clue to the deformity he constantly battled.

It was painful for my mother to hear Dr. Carlson diagnose Elliott as an "ataxia" type of spastic, but he ended his evaluation with the words that she had come to Florida to hear. "There's a chance that Elliott will eventually be able to walk. He could learn to talk, and someday he might very well attend normal schools, even college, if he

44

so desires. Consequently, Mrs. Weiss, I'm pleased to tell you that we can accept Elliott for our nursery program."

My mother was ecstatic. At that instant, and all of her doubts vanished. Whatever the cost, my parents would scrape it together; whatever the burden, they would share it. The loss of their precious child's company at home, not seeing his beautiful smile, not feeling the warmth of his loving arms, as dear as these tender moments are to young parents with their first child, all seemed a small price to pay for the chance that Elliott could learn to walk and talk and mature into a normal young man.

"I imagine this will mean some hardship on your part," Dr. Carlson said.

"I understand," my mother agreed. "I don't want to give up on Elliott, not if you can do something for him... " She was willing to sacrifice anything, even if it meant a painful separation from her beloved son.

"I think we can do a great deal for him. We're not like most institutions that deal with the handicapped. Our purpose goes beyond keeping the children occupied. We attempt to give them all of the education they are capable of absorbing, and all of the physical ability that is possible for them. We have to develop their concentration, perseverance, and ability if they are ever to overcome their handicap and adjust to their environment as contributing members of society."

"And when I speak of hardship for you, I don't necessarily mean the hardship of separation, or of the somewhat considerable cost of maintaining Elliott in this program. I mean that you must, in your own contacts with Elliott, maintain the same strict regimen that he will face here."

"From my own experience, and from the things that I have seen here, I know that many parents and teachers make too many concessions to the handicapped. This is unfair to them because if

45

we make things too easy, these children never develop the ability
to fight their affliction. Instead, the spastic may develop behavioral
dysfunctions that make it difficult, if not impossible, to conform to
normal standards. And that, of course, is our ultimate goal, to make
your son as normal as possible."

"While he is here, he will be subjected to rigid discipline and
strict routine. These methods result in much more rapid improvement
than leniency and compassion."

My mother's entire body went weak at the words. She had
to bring her handkerchief from her purse and dab her eyes before she
could reply. "Doctor, let's do whatever it takes. I don't know how to
thank you enough."

He waited patiently while she composed herself and then
continued.

"It won't be easy, Mrs. Weiss, but I think Elliott has come to
us in time. Early treatment of this problem is essential. Even now, he
must unlearn the motion habits he has developed. He must be taught
to use his body correctly. With ataxia, this is a particularly difficult
problem because the individual does not always have a clear idea of
what his limbs are doing. There seems to be a gap in the path that the
brain uses to get messages to and from the arms and legs. We have to
develop new pathways for these messages to travel."

"We also need to begin immediate work on his personality
development. At his age, he is already developing the character traits
that will individualize him throughout his life. Unless these traits are
carefully shaped through discipline and reward, the spastic individual
may easily become neurotic or even psychotic. We must make certain
that this does not happen to your son."

Dr. Carlson leaned forward across his desk, engrossed in what
he was saying, although he must have lectured a thousand mothers in
the same manner over the years. My mother could hear the conviction

46

ringing in his voice and she concentrated to absorb everything he was telling her.

"The greatest barrier to the treatment of children with cerebral palsy is the lack of self-discipline. They develop highly fluctuating emotions, from extreme depression to euphoria. When we examined Elliott today, he was in an excitable state. We expected this because the surroundings are unfamiliar to him. We have to gain his confidence before he can progress."

"Many times, when I see our children feeding and dressing themselves or learning to walk on crutches, I can't help thinking about the state they were in when their parents brought them to see me for the first time. We have to tame their excitability, for they can only progress in a calm, quiet atmosphere."

"What we will be doing for the next few weeks is getting Elliott to work with our therapists. They have all been carefully chosen for their ability to work with handicapped children. Too often, when a parent tries to teach a child to walk or talk, he or she may show too much anxiety over the child's progress, and the child becomes excitable and unmanageable as a reflection of this anxiety. Discipline is the answer. We will get him to relax, we will get him to concentrate, and then, Mrs. Weiss, we will get him to walk."

"Just tell me what to do," said my mother.

He smiled with satisfaction and stood up, and again she marveled at his mobility and vigor in spite of his handicap.

"Right now, all I need you to do is go home and try not to worry. We'll take care of your son. If you like, I can have one of the attendants show you around the school before you leave. I think you will understand that your son will be in a very positive environment."

The Carlson School was, indeed, beautiful. It was situated on a beautiful section of rambling beachfront property that might have been mistaken for a luxurious tourist hotel. The building was of the

47

typical Mediterranean style that had become popular in South Florida. It had a red barrel-tiled roof and arched doorways hinting of Moorish origins. On the eastern side of the building a white strand of beach was bordered by palm trees and sea-grape trees stretching for miles in either direction, all of this in an area once reserved for millionaire vacationers.

Inside were spacious hallways with high ceilings and beautiful chandeliers. The severely handicapped children were housed in ground floor rooms while the others lived upstairs. Areas for speech, occupational and physical therapy, as well as formal schoolrooms were held in what obviously had been the drawing rooms and parlors of a magnificent estate.

There were about 60 residents at the school at that time. Most of them were even more severely handicapped than Elliott. My mother didn't question this, or the fact that the school was located between the two most prestigious East Coast resorts of the era. It was symbolic of Dr. Carlson's personal success, and she would only have the best for her child. In 1940, the $160 monthly tuition was an overwhelming sum, but Elliott needed a chance in life, and, if they had to, they would buy it for him.

"Ideally, we would like to keep Elliott for a year," Dr. Carlson said as he saw me out. "After that, as I've explained, there's a good chance he'll be ready to go home and take up a relatively normal existence. In some cases, however, we need to keep the child longer, sometimes for a lifetime. All I can promise is that we'll do what's best for Elliott."

During this conversation, Elliott was waiting with the attendants by the door. My mother knelt beside him, her hands cold and sweaty and my legs trembling. He smiled at her and he hugged her tightly with his feeble arms. She was barely able to find her voice. She felt he somehow knew that she was going to be leaving without him.

"Goodbye, Elliott. Be a good boy for the nice people here."

She held him tightly, refusing to let go until one of the attendants gently touched her shoulder. She drew back slowly and they took Elliott away, pushing him down the hallway in his stroller. And then he was gone.

She left the school, but was reluctant to go too far. Tillie and Julius were, as always, open in their hospitality, and she decided to remain in Florida so that she could visit Elliott. During the next few weeks, she visited the school frequently. Elliott seemed happy and well cared for, and he was adjusting rapidly. He was, in fact, making his first friends. He had never had true companionship, but here, with others similarly afflicted, he could be treated as an equal and communicate with children his own age. What we found even more encouraging in the first few weeks was that Elliott had begun to utter clear syllables and was beginning to string them together into coherent words.

Elliott's progress seemed miraculous, but when my mother returned home with Tillie and Julius, there was a great void in the household. She missed her son.

"I wouldn't worry, Rose," Tillie told her. "Eddie needs you back home, and Elliott has us here to look after him. We'll visit him every Sunday and take him on rides, buy him ice cream, show him he's still loved. Things couldn't be better."

She couldn't hide the eagerness in her voice. She was getting Elliott after all. My mother couldn't resent them for loving her son, but the situation was disconcerting nonetheless. Tillie would be a part-time parent by proxy and my mother would be returning home alone.

Elliott couldn't have more loving parents. How could my mother travel a thousand miles away and leave Elliott there? It just didn't seem right to her.

"Think of Eddie, home alone," Julius offered. "You know he married you for your cooking, Rose. The poor man is probably wasting away on canned food."

That, at least, brought a smile to her face. It was true. My father hated to cook and he hated going out to restaurants. My mother felt that she was neglecting him, but he had managed for 30 years before he'd gotten his live-in chef. Elliott had never been alone before.

"At least he'll be coming up to Long Island this summer," she rationalized. "That's not too far to visit."

"Of course not," Julius said beaming. "You can come see us next winter."

And so she left them and her son and went back to the cold North. My father was delighted with her return.

But without Elliott the house seemed empty. Each time my mother passed his room with the new bed and matching chest of drawers, each time she looked at the colorful hooked rug with the dog in the center, a rug she had made especially for Elliott's room, tears came to her eyes. She cried a lot during the next few months, tears that only a mother's heart can know. But she found solace and strength in telling herself that this was the only way her child could be helped.

Aunt Tillie and Uncle Julius visited Elliott faithfully each Sunday afternoon while he was in Pompano Beach. They wrote often, describing how Elliott anxiously awaited them, not budging from the lobby sofa until they arrived.

Every Sunday meant love and affection for Elliott: hugs, kisses, a ride in the car, and a not-to-be-missed ice cream treat. They sent my parents many pictures showing Elliott's developing maturity.

One day the school informed my parents that a local carpenter had constructed a large wooden walker for Elliott. "It's sort of box-shaped, rectangular, and has bars on each side," the letter said. "Elliott is using the walker to give him support, and he pushes it along the sidewalks to make his daily rounds of the school." Pictures of Elliott and the walker were enclosed in the letter. They also learned that if he couldn't make it go fast enough to suit him, he would simply crawl out of it and scamper about on his hands and knees.

"In no time he'll be able to take care of himself, and you and I can get on with our life together," My father assured my mother.

"But what kind of life is it if we have to abandon Elliott?"

"We haven't abandoned him, Rose. It's just for a little while."

But my mother couldn't cast away the doubts. Instead she found herself pacing the living room floor, wringing her hands, wondering how Elliott was doing. The letters from the school were encouraging, but she wondered how much they were self-serving and how much they really reflected Elliott's contentment.

My father returned from the pharmacy one night to find my mother standing in the nursery, staring at Elliott's things, fighting tears for the thousandth time. He put his arm around her.

"I thought we might go out to dinner tonight. You can use a night away from the dishes."

"I had to use the house money for the rent, Eddie," my mother told him. "There's a casserole in the oven."

"In that case a casserole will be fine. We can go for a nice walk after dinner."

"I don't feel like walking, Eddie." She took a last look around Elliott's bedroom and then went into the kitchen to sit down at the table. My father followed her.

"Rose, you're going to have to snap out of it. You can't have Elliott and help him at the same time. We're doing what's best for him."

51

"It's not fair, Eddie. It's not what I wanted our life to be like."

The tears were gushing now, and she put her head in her hands to hide them while her back was racked with sobs. My father watched for a moment, and she could sense his body tensing without having to look at him.

"Rose, we can't go on like--" he started, and then stopped so sharply, my mother looked up at him. He was clutching his stomach with a look of disgust on his face. He whirled away from her and hurried into the bathroom. Alarmed, she ran after him and got there just in time to see him pour a spoonful of his medicine from the cabinet and swallow it.

"Eddie, are you all right?"

He capped the bottle, not looking at her.

"Elliott's going to be all right, Rose. We're going to keep on doing for him like we've been doing. We'll go to the bank tomorrow and get a loan so we can afford to get by for now."

"Eddie, we don't need a loan. We can find other ways to save. I'm shopping the bargains now, and I stay out of the department stores so I won't buy anything. We can skip the dinners and the movies, and we really don't need any more clothes. Maybe we can save enough to go see Elliott..."

My father was staring at my mother. He took a deep breath and then nodded.

"I'll try keeping the store open until nine, Rose. Maybe it will help. You can't deny yourself everything for Elliott's sake."

"But I will, Eddie, especially if it means I can see him."

He hugged her. "Rose, you love him so much."

She squeezed him back, grateful that he understood. When they finally separated, he tapped her on the chin affectionately.

"Are you sure you don't want to go for a walk with me tonight?"

"Maybe later," she said. "I'm putting together a care package and a letter for Elliott. When that's done, I'll walk with you if there's still time."

"Sure, Rose," he said. "I understand. We'll walk when you get that done."

By the time she was done with her letter and had sealed the box she was sending to Florida, she was ready for a short walk, but by that time, my father had got to bed and had fallen asleep.

Elliott liked the Carlson School. His bed was along the wall of his room and there was a window above it where he could look out and see the birds. There were seagulls and pelicans and mockingbirds. He had a net, like a hammock, that was strung the length of the bed, and he had all his stuff in it—his clothes and books and everything. But he dreaded some of the things they made him do at the school. The staff was very tough on him, except for one. Ed Wobloscky was becoming a second father to Elliott. He was wonderful. Ed would take a horse cart and they would ride up and down the beach. They had a great time together.

"Elliott is so precious," Tillie wrote. "He knows that Sunday is the day we go to see him, and I don't know what he would ever do if we were forced to miss a trip. When we arrive, he is always sitting on the sofa in the lobby waiting for us. They've told us that sometimes he has waited almost an hour, but he won't budge if he knows we're coming."

"He's so much better than the other children at the school. Some of them are so pitiful, hardly able to do anything for themselves. But then there are many others who get around on crutches, or with braces, or sometimes without any help at all. I'm sure that's the way it will be with Elliott."

"He loves our visits because he knows they mean hugs and kisses and affection. He needs that after the routine of the school. He

53

can't wait to get in the car for his Sunday drive. We take him to an ice cream parlor by the beach and he always has a big sundae. The people in the parlor know him now and are always very nice to him. It's so wonderful. I hope you're not worrying about him, because he really is in good hands."

That year, Dr. Carlson engaged a special train to take the children from Florida to East Hampton so they could travel in private- -away from the cruel stares of other children and adults. He had established his Long Island school in an old estate similar to the one in Pompano Beach. It stood on a wooded site next to the breeze swept dunes of the southern coastal beach, where students could continue exercising in the ocean and enjoy the open air.

"Elliott is beginning to pronounce many words," the school told my mother. "He is making sentences and we can understand them. His coordination is much improved. In occupational therapy, he is learning to string wooden beads and to work with the pegboard. This helps him develop hand-eye coordination by requiring him to place square pegs in square holes, etc. While this is a simple task for a "normal" child, it is a significant accomplishment for Elliott."

"The children swim daily, weather permitting, and always under strict supervision. Elliott seems to be very happy with his surroundings; he is cooperative and his personality continues to be bright and cheerful, as you will see from the enclosed photographs."

The picture showed him playing on the beach with the other children and moving about the sidewalks in his walker. He was smiling in each picture. His legs seemed longer, and he was a great deal leaner. He looked like a beautiful young man, and from the pictures it was difficult to tell that he had any problems.

"Elliott's third birthday was a special event," another letter informed my parents. "We had a party for him on September 8th, complete with a chocolate cake and six candles—three for good luck."

"In addition, as you will see in the attached photo, Elliott has had his first professional haircut. We think you will agree he looks very handsome." Her boy's baby curls were gone, replaced by an attractive crew cut. He looked like any other youngster ready to try out for Little League.

In physical therapy, Elliott was taking special daily sessions along parallel bars designed to help him develop greater control of his leg muscles. He wore high brown shoes for extra support, and he was learning how to lace and tie them. They purchased special clothing for him—pullover shirts, and trousers and underwear with elastic waistbands. In what seemed like no time at all, he was learning to dress himself.

"This is all very encouraging," said a letter from the school. "While we realize the development he has shown has taken some time, we feel that Elliott can continue to progress. We are returning to Pompano Beach shortly, and we hope you will permit us to keep Elliott with us for at least another year. We believe we can have him walking by then."

My mother found the letter opened on the table when she came home from visiting friends at midday. She read it with a sinking feeling, knowing that they wanted to keep her apart from her son for another year. The time had already seemed so long, and after all, how much of his progress could have been accomplished at home, surrounded by the love and affection of his family?

She wondered why my father had happened to be home before noon to open the letter. She looked around the living room curiously and then went to the bedroom door. My father was undressed and lying under the covers asleep. Alarmed, she hurried over to his side and rashly awakened him.

"Eddie, what's wrong?"

He shook off his sleep slowly, and when he looked at her he

seemed weaker than she'd ever seen him.

"I didn't feel well, Rose. I had to come home." His voice was barely a whisper.

"Do you want me to call Dr. Craft? Who's taking care of the store?"

"I already saw him. He told me to close up the store and come home to lie down."

"What's wrong? Is it the flu? Should I get you some chicken soup?" "I couldn't keep down breakfast again," he said.

"Again?"

"I've been feeling weak and my stomach has been cramping on me. Dr. Craft wants to run some tests, but he thinks it's a duodenal ulcer. He gave me some more medicine."

"He *thinks*? Eddie, you know how he was with Elliott. Maybe we should take you somewhere else to get checked. We can't afford to mess around with this. Maybe it's something serious."

"Rose, this time he's right." My father tried to make his voice stronger, and just barely succeeded. "And an ulcer *is* serious. He says if I keep on with this pressure, my condition will only get worse. He thinks that it might be a good idea if we didn't keep the store."

My mother sat down on the chair beside the bed.

"Eddie, what would we do? How will we afford to live?"

"We'd find a way to make do. Did you see the letter from Elliott's school?"

"Eddie, how can we keep him in school another year if you can't work?"

"I was thinking about it before you came home, Rose. What I really need is time to relax. The climate is bad for me here. Maybe we should both go to Florida for a while."

My feelings of impending tragedy immediately disappeared.

"Eddie, that would be perfect! We could stay with Tillie and

Julius until you got better. Maybe you could open a store down there."

"Maybe we could. I'd have to pass the Florida pharmaceutical boards first, but they can't be any tougher than the ones here. Besides, I know a thing or two more about mixing potions than the kids coming fresh out of the University of Florida. I'd enjoy being close to Elliott down there and I know you'd feel better if you could see him more often."

"Oh, Eddie, let's do it!" My mother said. "I'll write Tillie and Julius right away. Do you think it will take long to sell the store?"

"The people from a chain in Pittsburgh have been wanting to get hold of it. I think we can make a deal that will keep us going for a while."

My mother was thrilled about the possibility of moving to Florida, but she was worried about my father's health. The strain of putting up a strong front for my mother had been wearing away at him. All this time he had been worried about Elliott, about my mother, about the store, and about paying their bills. And he had been trying to be so strong.

It would be better now. It really would. My mother could see Elliott whenever she wanted. He would know that his parents were still there for him and that they still loved him.

Much to my mother's surprise, however, Tillie's reply to her letter seemed strangely
formal:

"Dear Rose, of course we will be happy to have you and Eddie stay with us until you establish yourselves here. We will make up the spare bedroom again. Julius and I will be glad to accompany you whenever you wish to visit Elliott in Pompano. Sincerely, Aunt Tillie."

"That's an awfully short letter for your aunt," my father said. "Are you sure she doesn't think we're imposing?"

"No, not Tillie. She wouldn't dream of having us stay anywhere else. I think she's a little disappointed that she won't have Elliott to herself this year."

My mother felt triumphant when she said it, in spite of herself. Elliott had to know who his mother was. If he was going to succeed, and mature, she wanted to be a major part of it.

As my father had predicted, the Pittsburgh company was eager to get the store and they made a good settlement for it. My mother soon found herself packing up their belongings and making preparations to leave the house where they had stayed since the day they were married—the house where Elliott was born.

My mother waited on the sidewalk while my father closed up the store for the last time and handed the keys to one of the men from Pittsburgh. They shook hands, both of them smiling and laughing, but when my father walked away he looked pale. He stopped on the curb and took a last, long look at the front door of his business.

"It'll be all right," my mother told him, squeezing his arm.

He nodded, silent, and opened the car door for her. He paused another moment before walking around to the driver's seat, and when he slid behind the wheel he took a long, deep breath.

"You're not feeling ill, are you, Eddie?" My mother asked him.

He turned the key in the ignition and put the car in gear, but he waited before driving away. My father seemed to need a final look at his store before answering. "I'm just a little tired, Rose," he said softly.

That night, my father went to bed early, but he slept fitfully. Then he was up by 4:30 a.m., checking the house a final time for any forgotten items, and then he carefully stowed all their worldly goods into the car and trailer. My mother heard him moving about and got up to put on the coffee while he was taking a load of cartons downstairs, but the coffee pot and the coffee were already gone. She stood helplessly in her housecoat in the middle of the kitchen, wondering how she could prepare his breakfast so that he would have the strength for the drive. When he came in he knew immediately what she was thinking.

"We'll stop on the highway," he said. "It's good to have an early start."

She got dressed quickly and packed her housecoat into the suitcase. The closets were emptied, and the house looked as deserted as it had felt in the long months of their son's absence. They stopped at the threshold on the way out and looked around, trying to engrave the last view of it in their minds.

"It's good to leave," my father said. "There has been so much sadness and worry here."

"But there were good times, too, Eddie. Lots of them."

"We'll have plenty more," he said, and he escorted my mother out the door to the car. The sun was coming up through the full leaves of the oak trees in the yard as they pulled out of the driveway and turned south. My mother told herself she wasn't going to look back, but she looked out the back window anyway until she could no longer see their home. She felt as if she was leaving part of her soul there, abandoned.

They drove down through the mountains to Cumberland and then followed the narrow Blue Ridge Highway south. In those days, interstate travel was a series of narrow roads and endless small towns. They had the usual tourist trepidations as they crossed the Mason-Dixon Line into Dixie, where every Northerner still imagined lingering Confederate provincialism and bigotry.

"Don't drive too fast, Eddie," my mother cautioned. "They'll see the Pennsylvania license plate and give you a ticket if you're not careful."

"I'm careful, Rose," he said. "I've done this before, you

know?"

"I just want you to be careful, that's all."

My father laughed at my mother, and then they enjoyed the scenery for the first few hundred miles. As the strain of the drive began to wear on him, however, he talked less frequently. My mother could see his jaw set and his body become more rigid as he held the wheel. She wished that she had learned to drive so that she could relieve him for part of the journey. But there had never been much need for her to drive.

My mother dozed occasionally when the monotony of the journey began to wear on her. During the first day's travel, my father indulged my mother by stopping to let her look at scenery and small roadside attractions, but by the afternoon of the second day, he even wanted to avoid the rest stops. "Let's just get there already," he kept saying.

At night, in the motels, he tossed in his sleep, and my mother could hear him muttering wordless sentences in his dreams. He would get up several times during the night and head into the bathroom, where he would stay for a long time.

The temperature grew increasingly warm as they headed south. Their car was not air conditioned, and my mother could see the heat was starting to take its toll on my father. Sweat beaded on his forehead, and his face was becoming paler and paler. Now my father scarcely spoke to my mother at all, and he looked increasingly impatient when she said anything. But she could hardly keep still as she grew more and more excited with every mile they traveled closer to their destination.

"I'm sure the school will let me bring Elliott home now and then for vacations," said my mother. "We can take him to the beach again, Eddie. When we get a house, let's make sure that it's close to the beach. I like Coral Gables, if we can afford it. There are lots of

60

nice old houses there that shouldn't cost very much. I was thinking about a duplex. We could live in one side and rent the other, using the rent money to pay off the mortgage. That way it would hardly cost anything. If you like, when we get there..."

And then she realized that the car was slowing down. My father pulled off to the side, very slowly, and when they came to a complete stop, he closed his eyes and leaned his head against the steering wheel.

"Eddie, what is it?"

"I just need a minute to rest, Rose. Just be quiet a minute."

My father was taking long, deep breaths, each one getting longer. Suddenly, he flung open the door, scrambled behind the car, and began retching violently onto the sandy shoulder. My mother rushed to help support him. At first he tried to wave her off, but as a new wave of nausea overcame him he clutched tightly to her support.

"Eddie. . . . "

But he had dry heaves and couldn't answer. My mother looked around, frightened. A brownish-yellow plain surrounded them on all sides, broken only by scrub palmetto, pine trees, and cattle. The highway was an empty expanse of asphalt stretching interminably into the distance.

"Eddie, please, what can I do?"

He finally caught his breath and my mother helped him lean against the car. His skin was strangely cold, yet damp to the touch. Perspiration darkened his entire shirt.

"I'll be all right, Rose," he swore. "Just a little car sick."

"Eddie, you were never car sick when you were driving. You need to see a doctor."

"I'll see one in Miami, Rose. We'll make it. Just let me rest a while."

Against my mother's better judgment, she let him go to sleep in the car. It was close to noon and the heat was becoming unbearable. She was certain that whatever was wrong with my father, sleeping in that oven wasn't going to help him. She rolled down all the windows and opened the doors on the passenger's side to let in as much breeze as possible, and then she stood outside the car, frantic, wondering what to do next. Every time a car passed, she wondered if she should stop it and ask them to send for help. Three cars finally did stop, but each time she wavered, sure that my father would be angry with her if she did anything. She assured them that everything was all right and sent them on their way.

She kept checking to make certain my father was breathing all right. His skin seemed to be burning, but she told herself that it was just the heat of the car's interior. Finally, about three o'clock in the afternoon, he woke up and sat upright behind the steering wheel. She looked at him with trepidation.

"Let's get started," he said, turning on the ignition.

"Eddie, let's stop somewhere close by. It's not too late to have someone look at you today."

He wasn't listening. He pulled onto the highway with exaggerated slowness.

"It's OK now. I'm rested. Let's just get there."

It was four more hours before they pulled up in front of the house in Miami. Julius and Tillie came out laughing and smiling, with arms spread to greet us, but their faces quickly took on a look of concern when they saw my father's condition.

He could barely walk. Julius quickly put an arm around him and helped him toward the house. Halfway to the door, my father's legs buckled and he nearly fell down. Julius regained his balance and guided my father through the front door.

"Rose, how could you let him drive like that?" Tillie demanded. "What's wrong with him?"

"I don't know," I said, hurrying after my husband. "We have to find a doctor for him. Tillie, I'm scared."

"Tillie, I really appreciate your offer to let us stay with you and Julius again, but I think it would be better if we rented a room closer to the hospital. Eddie is seeing so many doctors and the traveling back and forth is not good for him."

"I understand, Rose, but if you should change your mind, both of you are more than welcome to stay with us," Tillie replied.

"Mr. Weiss, I'm, sorry to say this, but the tests show you have an ulcer and your appendix is on the verge of perforating. The only cure is surgery as quickly as possible," said Dr. Hanson.

"Doctor, he will be all right, won't he?" My mother said, searching for assurance.

"Yes, Mrs. Weiss, he'll be fine. Your husband will be in the intensive care unit for a few days and then in a regular ward for about ten days. After that, he can go home."

My father's surgery lasted about two hours, although it felt like two years to my mother. Finally, the doctor came out to see her.

"Mrs. Weiss, your husband is in the recovery room and doing well," the doctor told her.

After fourteen days in the hospital, m father came home and my mother gave him all the loving care she could to get him back onto his feet. Once he started to feel better, he began to study for the Florida Pharmaceutical Examination. My mother knew he was worried about something, but he had been a pharmacist for a long time, so she knew it wasn't about the exam.

"Eddie, what's wrong?" My mother asked. "You seem preoccupied about something and it can't be the exam, because I know you'll have no problems there," my mother said one evening.

"We've spent just about all of our savings from the sale of the pharmacy and I haven't been able to buy another one here in Miami

Beach. What are we going to do when the money runs out?"

"Eddie, I've been worried about the money too, but we've always done okay and I'm sure that in the future we'll be just fine. All you have to do is pass the examination and then you can focus more attention on starting up your own business here."

Two weeks later they were on their way to Gainesville. My father passed his examination without any problems, but instead of going back to Miami, he suggested they head back to Pennsylvania for a while.

My mother wasn't happy about this decision, especially given what they'd gone through leaving California, PA and moving to Florida, but he'd been so ill; he needed her and she couldn't say no to him.

After a couple of weeks in Pennsylvania, my father came home happier than she'd seen him in a long time.

"Rose, I found a pharmacy for sale here in town that we can afford. I want to buy it so that we can get back on our feet again," he said.

She had hoped that this stay in Pennsylvania would be short-lived and that they would soon go back to Elliott, but once again she couldn't say no. My father was so positive and happy.

February of 1942 marked Elliott's second full year with Dr. Carlson. That month they received a letter from the school suggesting they take Elliott home and enroll him in a kindergarten for normal youngsters in preparation for entrance into public school.

Progress had been slow. Elliott could dress himself and he seemed to have better control of his muscles, but he still could not walk independently. Nevertheless, Dr. Carlson believed he should be home with my parents and exposed to normal children for emotional reasons.

The letter, combined with the numbing cold of the Pennsylvania winters, and with my mother's loneliness, would help them make a decision.

"Eddie," my mother shouted as she rushed into the store, "Elliott can come home and we can be a family again."

My father's face showed relief. Finally, his son was making progress, and maybe soon they would be a normal family.

"There's a problem though, Eddie," my mother said.

"What now, Rose," he replied.

"It will soon be winter here and Elliott is not used to the cold and damp anymore. I think I should go back to Florida and get a house down there. You could visit us and see the progress he is making."

She could see from the look on my father's face that he was not happy with this idea.

"Eddie, we've come so far with Elliott," She said. "Why destroy all of his progress now?"

"OK, Rose, you go to Florida and I'll stay here and keep the business going. I'll visit you when I can," he said resignedly.

Once again, my mother found herself back on the train to Florida. This time, her son would be back home with her. When she arrived, she rented a unit in a small duplex, brought Elliott home from Dr. Carlson's, and called Sarah, the nurse who had been with her at his birth.

"Sarah," she said. "Elliott is home and I will need some help taking care of him. Can you come and stay with me? I'll pay you fifteen dollars a week plus room and board."

"I'll be there in a couple of hours," she said. "I'd love to help you with Elliott." Sarah also agreed to go to Dr. Carlson's with my mother to observe the therapy treatments so that they would know how to continue them on their own. However, she didn't know how soon Sarah's generosity would end.

"Elliott, you're going to school today," my mother told him. "You will be with other little boys and girls your age. Isn't that exciting?"

He laughed with delight. At least now, maybe, he would have friends.

But when she took Elliott to the school the principal said, "I'm sorry, Mrs. Weiss, but Elliott's attention span does not allow him to do the things the other children are doing and he gets very disruptive. I'm very sorry," he added.

"Don't worry, Mrs. Weiss," Sarah said. "Maybe if I stay at the school with him, he'll be better."

"That's a good idea, Sarah. I'm sure they won't mind you being there to help."

Once again, my mother heard the same story from the principal. The only time Elliott behaved in class was when Sarah was with him. Otherwise, he distracted the other children. And when it came time for the children's rest period, he wouldn't leave them alone. My mother noticed he was becoming more and more emotionally disturbed. She was sure that Elliott was acting out his frustrations over not being able to do the things the other children were doing.

My mother tried one more time at a different kindergarten, with Sarah taking care of Elliott at the school, which was run by two middle-aged ladies who liked Sarah.

"I'm sorry, Mrs. Weiss," Sarah said one day, "but they have offered me one hundred dollars a week to go work for them full-time."

"Please, Sarah, stay and help me with Elliott," my mother pleaded. "You know how fond he is of you. You can do so much with him."

My mother decided now was time to purchase a small pair of adjustable wooden crutches. Each afternoon Sarah and my mother spent time with Elliott in the front yard trying to get him to take a few

66

steps. Although the crutches had foam-rubber pads, he complained of pain constantly. "They hurt me here," he said, pointing under his arms in defiance of the crutches and, perhaps, of the world.

He tried again to take one step, then flung the crutches in the air screaming, "They hurt my arms, they hurt my arms!"

That usually ended their efforts for the day. Meanwhile, Elliott was taking swimming lessons at the Venetian Pool, a large, beautiful public swimming facility in Coral Gables. Realistically, Sarah and my mother didn't expect him to learn to swim, but we were certain that the lessons would give him additional assurance and helped to strengthen his leg muscles, which he needed to walk. My mother continued to hope.

Meanwhile, this was the spring of 1942, the nation was at war, and the streets of Miami were filled with the bobbing caps of servicemen. My father came to visit as Elliott was recovering from an uncomplicated bout with the mumps. My father enjoyed the respite from work, and it wasn't long before Elliott resumed his outdoor activities.

They all gathered in the yard after lunch and my mother said, "Show daddy how nicely you've learned to walk on your crutches, Elliott. Go ahead, show daddy."

Elliott peered at my father, Sarah, and then at my mother. For a minute he appeared quite serious. Then he replied, "OK, I'll walk for daddy."

Together we gazed intently while Elliott put his crutches in place. Then, to our utter disbelief, he proceeded to walk around the house with the aid of his crutches! He stumbled, his movements were not smooth, but he was walking--albeit on crutches. Yes, clumsily, unsteadily, not well-balanced, but joyfully, he was walking! After countless exercises, incessant prodding, daily encouragement, and the determination of a brave little boy, Elliott was indeed walking.

"I can't believe it," my father said.

"Look at him!" Sarah shouted.

"That's a good boy, Elliott," my mother shouted. "That's wonderful."

My parents sat together outside, long after Elliott and Sarah had gone to bed. Today had been a milestone. Words were not necessary. Our youthful joys of marriage had matured after all we had been through together, and now, on the quiet evening of this eventful day, they shared a real joy. We had courage for the future, wherever it would lead. Although we did not talk about our feelings often, we were always working together toward the goal of Elliott's happiness.

Then my father returned to Pennsylvania, and my mother was left to care for Elliott. One of the hardest things at that time was the coldness Elliott was experiencing from the other children. My mother bought ice cream, candy, cookies, and, in fact, everything children love to eat, all in the hopes that they would come play with Elliott. Unfortunately, none of it worked and Elliott remained a lonely little boy.

Then one day in September of 1942, she received a letter informing her that her mother had suffered a severe stroke and was dying. She had to leave for West Virginia immediately.

My mother called Sarah. "Would you please take care of Elliott while I'm gone? He knows you, and I don't have anyone else to leave him with," she said.

"Don't worry," she replied. "I'll take care of him."

As it turned out, she arrived in West Virginia in time for her mother's funeral. Afterwards, she decided to go to Pennsylvania to see my father for a short time.

When I returned to Miami, my mother went to pick up Elliott at Sarah's house.

"I'm sorry, Mrs. Weiss," Sarah told me. "Elliott isn't feeling very well."

Elliott was as jaundiced as he was when he was a baby. It turned that she had been feeding him a largely vegetarian diet, and it wasn't agreeing with him. Fortunately, it wasn't anything serious, and Elliott was soon back to normal once my mother took him home and returned him to his usual diet. Less than two weeks later, my mother had good news for Elliott: "Daddy is coming home to live with us."

My father had called with the news that he had sold the new pharmacy and was now moving to South Florida for good.

In order for Elliott to be exposed to a normal educational environment and to other children, my mother did extensive research into private kindergartens. She was asked to remain in the classroom with Elliott for a while to see if he could adjust to the class before a permanent arrangement could be determined. These people did not have the faintest idea what cerebral palsy was, and they did not seem interested in learning about the disability. Elliott was not classified as a normal student. He constantly shifted in his seat, determined to get up and wander around. Not surprisingly, Elliott did not stay long at any of the schools. The teachers were not patient and their attitude reflected this feeling. As a result, the weekly tuition was being wasted. My mother became discouraged and decided to keep Elliott at home for a while. She purchased some books to work with him on his own level, and let him play with Mary Ann, the little girl who lived next door.

Twice a week, my mother once again took Elliott, who was now about five years old, to the Venetian Pool for swimming lessons. Although he never mastered the techniques of the strokes, the exercise was good for strengthening his muscles.

Their friends, Bill and Lil Kotler, often came to take Elliott on outings, as well as to take my mother shopping. Bill, a self-employed carpenter, would let Elliott watch him make things. One item was a large wooden stroller for Elliott so that my mother could take him for long walks through the neighborhood because Elliott couldn't cover any long distances on his crutches.

Mary Ann's mother was very understanding and kind-hearted. She encouraged her daughter to play with Elliott. What a wonderful feeling to be accepted!

Around this time, my father's sisters, Esther and Sadie, wrote that they were coming to visit and to look for a home. Each had a child who would be ready for college the next year. They both quickly found homes close to where my parents lived, and then it wasn't long before other members of the Weiss family followed.

Later that summer, my father's brother Emil paid my parents a visit. He also wanted to relocate to Miami. Emil and my parents found a beautiful two-bedroom duplex across the street from Coral Way Elementary School, where they planned to enroll Elliott. The east side of the duplex was vacant, so Emil's family moved in, but my parents had to wait until the tenant's lease expired before they could move into their side of the duplex.

Shortly after their move, Emil and Essie divorced and left Miami. They rented their side to Peggy, the sister of the late Grace Kelly, Princess of Monaco, and her naval husband. My mother and Peggy became great friends. Peggy had a lot of patience with Elliott and gave him a lot of attention. Her schooling in the parochial school system taught her love and compassion for all mankind, including the disabled.

Whatever chore Peggy was engaged in, Elliott followed her. He would try to help her as much as he could, but she joked with him and took time out for a drink of Coke and cookies. Elliott would help her pull the weeds in the yard and would help her hang the laundry from the clothesline. Elliott and Peggy became such good pals, but then the Navy pulled all their forces out of Miami and they had to move back to Philadelphia. Then my parents and Elliott's days seemed so empty until it was time for Elliott to begin school again. My parents purchased a four-seater swing set and served refreshments in order to entice the neighborhood children use our yard as a playground, hoping that Elliott could make some friends. For a while, this seemed to be working out fine, but before the summer had ended, it was clear that the children were there for the free food and the new play equipment. When Elliott would go to their homes, he found that he was not welcome.

In September, the time came to register Elliott for first grade. Their beautiful new home, with its airy front screened porch and its many fruit trees, had taken on an air of excitement. They no longer had the financial worries of private schooling, and they now lived in a neighborhood with thirteen children about Elliott's age. Their luck had shifted, or so they thought. They truly believed the time was right for a new positive beginning at Coral Way Elementary, which was just cross the street from their new home.

If Elliott could find just one child who would become a real friend and companion, it would have meant so much to them. A whole new world would open up for him. But maybe that was too much for them to hope for.

Their next-door neighbors, Bob and Edie Schweitzer, had a son named Howie, who was one year younger than Elliott. At first the two boys played rather well together. Bob was still in the service, giving my parents a lot of time to spend together. They shared babysitting duties so they could each have a free evening one night per week. They also shared taking the boys with them on grocery trips.

However, for reasons they never fully understood, when Bob returned home the friendship between their families ceased, so Elliott and my mother kept busy with their own family. Aunt Tillie and Uncle Julius visited us often. They took them shopping and to places where they could see new and interesting things such as the shore in Miami Beach, the Crandon Park Zoo, and many of the other beautiful recreational areas in South Florida.

When registration day finally arrived, my parents walked Elliott to the school and waited in the registration line. Nervously, my mother crossed her fingers in hopes that all would go well. Elliott looked so handsome in his bright new shirt and pants, and in his beautiful new leather shoes, which she had shined to perfection. He had a big smile for his new teacher.

When it was finally my parent's turn they were greeted by the registrar; who quickly told them that they could not accept a child on crutches. He was considered handicapped and would have to attend a special school—the Roosevelt School for Exceptional Children—operated under the Dade County Public School System with grades one through seven. Another great disappointment had crushed their dreams that Elliott could finally fit into a mainstream educational program.

After calling the Roosevelt School that same day, my mother quickly learned the procedure. Elliott would be picked up by bus at 8:00 a.m. and would not be returned home until 4:00 p.m. A cafeteria would provide lunches, but in order to have breakfast at home and get dressed on time, my mother had to get Elliott up by 7:00 each morning. At this point, Elliott was wearing long braces prescribed by the Crippled Children's Society. They were strapped at the hips and ankles and required 20 minutes to adjust them to his body.

So when school started the next day, my mother woke Elliott up, helped him get dressed, put on his braces, and helped him with his bathroom business. By the time she'd seen him onto the school bus and placed his crutches underneath the seat, my mother was emotionally exhausted and physically drained. Life was getting crueler for them by the day. Their dream of Elliott going to school across the street from their new home had turned into a frustrating nightmare. They had chosen the ideal home and location but the wrong school!

Roosevelt School was a pink art deco building built in 1925. It had beautiful tile floors and its ceilings gave it a feeling of grandeur that often reminded my mother of the Carlson School in Pompano Beach. It was formerly a private club and had been purchased by the school board to be converted into a school for disabled children.

Fortunately, my father's health was improving, so he started to look for work, and before long he received a phone call from the Alton Road Pharmacy, a large, modern store in Miami Beach. He was interviewed, offered a job, and he promptly accepted.

The end of World War II signalled the return home of many servicemen and their families, bringing an influx of people to the Miami area. Thousands of servicemen from up north had trained in Miami Beach, and many decided to return when the war ended. In addition, many parents of discharged war veterans were among the new arrivals, causing the real estate market to flourish even more. Realtors would gather for lunch at the drug store where my father worked to discuss the numerous opportunities to buy and sell properties for a quick profit. My parents were lucky to get into some of those deals, and for a short while, they owned part of a hotel, an apartment house, and some commercial property. All of these investments were modest money-makers.

Saturday nights for my parents were usually busy. Their house was filled with relatives--usually Uncle Harry and Aunt Peppy, along with their daughters and their families. Sometimes they would play a game of poker. Elliott was so excited about family because they would always bring treats or games for him.

All the neighborhood children had tricycles or bicycles. To help him keep up with the other children, my parents purchased a bright red tricycle for Elliott, which he learned to ride immediately.

The school routine was new and the days were long, but Elliott seemed fascinated with going to the big white school and being in first grade. His excitement, however, was short-lived, for he soon discovered he was at school to learn and not to play. Elliott just did not relish sitting in his seat for any length of time, and he quickly learned that by raising his hand he could be excused to go to the bathroom. This became a frequent occurrence and the teacher finally requested that Elliott be examined by a doctor to rule out any kidney or bladder problems. Tests proved the problem wasn't medical. Their son simply could not apply himself. Fearing failure made it easier for him to avoid trying.

For the next two years, Elliott was kept in the first grade. None of his teachers had the "magic key" to unlock the door. "He seems to have it in him, but I don't know how to get it out of him," was how his teachers typically put it.

At the same time, Elliott was facing other problems; he was still finding it difficult to be accepted by the neighborhood children. His tricycle was good exercise for him and perhaps offered him a little more locomotion and independence than did his crutches. Elliott would speed around the block to visit the neighbors. My mother watched him struggle eagerly for friendship, yet he failed to find one real friend among the many children living in the area.

Why wasn't there just *one* child with the understanding to really like Elliott and have the patience to get to know him? Was it so difficult for another small child to realize how much Elliott needed another child's love and companionship? My mother learned very well how thoughtless and cruel normal children could be.

"You're crippled," a child would cry out to Elliott. Then Elliott would strike out at him with a crutch or simply run home in tears, hobbling furiously on both crutches.

74

Despite Elliott's speech and motor handicaps, Dr. Carlson had diagnosed his mentality as normal, and my mother was convinced that relationships with normal children would be important to his growth and maturity. My parents regularly invited children to their home, and many days they supposedly came over to play with Elliott in their large, screened-in porch. Elliott was eager for their companionship until they began to tease him.

One day my mother saw little Susie pick up a baseball and deliberately throw it at Elliott. It struck him in the center of his forehead. Quickly, my mother ran over and slapped Susie's hand, "Whatever do you mean hitting Elliott that way?" she scolded.

"Elliott's always kicking me, Mrs. Weiss," she said tearfully. "Sometimes I just can't stop from getting back at him." Immediately, my mother realized that she had been unfair to another child out of her pain for Elliott. She apologized to Susie and her mother.

Despite all the playground equipment in the backyard, the large assortment of toys, and the plentiful supply of cookies, candy, ice cream and drinks they purchased, they were not enough to buy the friendship of the other children. They finally decided friendship must come naturally or not at all. Sadly, those special childhood friendships never came.

Roosevelt School offered many facets for the disabled children. Physical, speech, and occupational therapies were offered on a weekly basis through the Crippled Children's Society. In the classroom, each teacher had about 15 students, so personal attention was impossible. Elliott's homeroom teacher reported, "He is overly emotional." Much to my parent's frustration, Elliott was developing the same psychological problems that Dr. Carlson had warned them about. But since Elliott's birth, there were no indications that he might suffer from mental deficiency. He smiled at 3 weeks old, laughed at 3 months old, and drank from a cup with some help at 8 months old, progressions comparable to other children his age.

On a positive note, they had a friendly neighbor, Fred. Fred had a lot of patience with Elliott and taught him many tricks about carpentry and camping. Fred often took his grandchildren camping and fishing, and to my parent's delight, he began to include Elliott on some of these trips. Fred was a sweet, retired gentleman who stayed at home a lot to work on his hobbies.

As soon as Elliott arrived home from school, he would head for Fred's house to see what he was making that day. Fred enjoyed the company and was glad to have an audience because his wife was often out or busy in the kitchen. Fred explained every carpentry tool and technique and he would often let Elliott try his skill at hammering nails. He showed him how to fold up a tent, and listed all the equipment they would need for each trip. The food supply was very important and he made a list of items that were needed from the market. He also taught Elliott about fishing. He explained the right kind of bait to use and what sort fish they were likely to catch.

One bright sunny day after Elliott got off the bus and had a drink of Coke, he went out to explore. This time it was a new adventure. About two hours had elapsed before my mother finally heard the familiar click of his crutches. Elliott had walked for the first time to Coral Way to visit Joe Toth, who ran a plant and nursery store. That was quite a hike for Elliott—the determining force to get there on his own was quite a milestone in his young life. He needed this confidence and he needed to communicate with someone he knew. He also needed to get there on his own legs. He made many trips after that first visit. Each time, Joe would call my mother and tell her Elliott had arrived and not to worry about him. She was pleased to know that they enjoyed each other's company.

Frances Huggins, the Roosevelt School principal, had a very active board of which my mother was a member. She was present at their annual Holiday Tea. The guest list included the mayor of Miami, principals of other schools, and other important members of the community. All holidays were heavily promoted to gain the public's attention, for Roosevelt was a special school, the only one of its kind in Miami. Mrs. Huggins was very devoted to the school and loved all her students.

Jane Collette, Elliott's first grade teacher, gave Elliott all satisfactory and even some excellent grades. In addition, he was making good progress in his physical activities. So how were my parents to know he wasn't learning anything? They were disillusioned by the fact that they had put forth so much effort to help their son, and good report cards made them believe that his years at the Roosevelt School were not fruitless. What was the major problem? Why didn't anyone have any answers?

After two years of frustration in the first grade, Elliott was refused a social promotion. My mother immediately wrote to Dr. Carlson, who agreed to re-enter him for another year in his program. That June, my parents flew Elliott to Dr. Carlson's school in East Hampton.

After analyzing the money involved in buying their home, the promising report cards, and teachers telling them how well Elliott was doing academically, my parents decided to sell the house and move back to Pennsylvania. Maybe their luck would change. Maybe Florida held bad promises for them. During their time there, they had found no answers--only mixed feelings.

But the wrath of the winter winds and the snows of Pennsylvania, combined with the separation from their son, depressed my parents. They prayed together each morning for a better life and a happy family, my father with his prayer book and my mother with her hands clasped. My father, with his happy memories of a large family and my mother with hers, longed for eventual stability in their family.

Once again, Elliott progressed at the Carlson School. A one-on-one basis always helped him to absorb and retain the knowledge that he was taught. Dr. Carlson could not understand why the teachers at Roosevelt could not reach him. "Either they are unqualified to teach special education or they just never took the time to understand the extent of Elliott's brain damage."

Along with the other students from the Carlson School, Elliott was transported to the Pompano Beach facility in the late fall. My parents were very anxious to see him again, to gaze at his boyish face and his beautiful smile, and to note how tall he had grown.

As my father continued to lose weight, his health problems increased, and my mother's nervous system suffered from all the emotional upsets they had experienced. My father blamed his physical problems on the emotional upsets, so he found a good doctor who helped get his nervous system in better shape. My parents decided it was time for a discussion about what direction to take and formulate some concrete plans for their future.

They decided that the time was right for them to drive back to Miami and purchase a new home that would also give them some income. My mother would look for work a few days per week. Luckily, they found a reliable real estate man, who found the ideal place for them on S.W. Sixth Street. The units in this pair of duplexes each had two bedrooms and a bath, a living and dining area, and a small back porch. It was ideal. They would live in one unit and rent out the others to help defray the expense of the school for the balance of the six months. Their hearts were full of great hopes with glowing reports of Elliott's progress in school. He was prepared for third grade and had high expectations for his future. Once again, they were on "cloud nine," but as usual, there were always more complications.

For starters, the two duplexes they purchased were filled with difficult tenants. Joe, who was a painter, gave them a worthless rent check, and then a few days later he moved out at midnight without notifying them. Isabelle, who lived in a front apartment, turned out to be a drug-addicted call girl. One evening one of her "customers" beat her up and my parents found her on the ground outside of her apartment bleeding and crying. They sent her to the hospital to get treatment.

With my father working, my mother was responsible for handling the rentals. It wasn't easy work. Their tenants came from all walks of life, and they quickly learned that this was a difficult way to acquire money.

In January, Elliott again joined them to live at home. It turned out that Dr. Carlson had over-evaluated Elliott, which is to say that he thought Elliott would eventually be mainstreamed and could even go to college someday. At this point, Dr. Carlson admitted that Elliott was no longer making any progress. This over-evaluation was due in part to Elliott's physical conditioning, which had surpassed that of most of his peers. As a result, Elliott would return to Roosevelt since that was the only school in the area in which he would be permitted to attend.

In the meantime, my mother's brother Bill, his wife Edith, and their daughter Marilyn had moved down from Charleston, West Virginia. They stayed with my parents for a few weeks until they found a home in Coral Gables. Then Bill opened a men's store, University Men's Shop, which included a tuxedo rental service. Elliott became attached to his Uncle Bill in a short period of time and called him frequently on the phone. Bill would kid him about helping out in the store when he got older, but Elliott took him seriously.

One Saturday Elliott was walking around outside and talking to the neighbors. My mother called him in for lunch. After calling his name several times with no response, she became worried. Elliott was nowhere to be seen. He had never strayed from home before. Her first thought was to call the police. She gave them a full description of Elliott and they promised to call her if he was found. To her relief, within half an hour she received a phone call. Elliott had been found at the bus station downtown and was being driven home.

His story was very interesting. He had wanted to go to Coral Gables to help his Uncle Bill in his store, but he didn't understand that bus fare was required in order to ride the bus. Even so, he did get onto a bus, but unfortunately, the bus he'd boarded was headed the wrong way. After a short talk, my mother helped Elliott to realize that what he'd done was wrong. Privately, however, my parents were happy because Elliott's desire to do something productive showed them his determination; they were convinced that with time and effort, Elliott might accomplish many things.

Ronnie and Al, my parent's tenants in their second apartment, were from Chicago. After a few months, their story about their severely retarded daughter unraveled. Their girl had been placed in an institution in their hometown because the medical reports indicated she could never learn anything and probably never walk or talk. She was considered a vegetable. Usually they did not tell anyone about Joanna, but after meeting Elliott, Ronnie chose to confide in my parents. Ronnie soon became pregnant and they looked forward to having a normal child. On schedule, Ronnie gave birth to a beautiful baby boy who became the light of their life, and consequently they moved to larger quarters.

Subsequently, Hansie, her mother, and her photographer husband, Werner, who was from Haiti, moved into the vacant apartment. Since Hansie and Werner both worked, Hansie's mother spent most of her time cooking and cleaning. My mother and her became good friends and she gave my mother some of her prized recipes from Europe. For Elliott's birthday, Werner insisted on taking some pictures of Elliott and presented them to my parents

80

as a gift. It was exciting for my parents to receive such a beautiful and professional gift. They all celebrated with birthday cake and ice cream.

While my father was working in Coral Gables, another real estate opportunity came my parent's way. It was an eight-unit apartment building in Coral Gables that housed naval servicemen.

In the fall, Elliott re-entered Roosevelt School in the third grade. He had learned to read, write, and do simple arithmetic, but academically, he was not willing to apply himself beyond that. In spite of the private tutoring he had received at Carlson, he was not doing his class work as quickly as the other children. His study habits were poor, and he had difficulty in accepting his responsibilities.

One report from a teacher, Eunice Kimbrough, stated, "Elliott has a very sweet, happy disposition and is a capable boy. However, he needs to learn to depend on himself and to develop a willingness to work. His short span of attention, his dependence, and his refusal to accept any personal responsibility are keeping his academic and social development at a very unsatisfactory level."

The following report noted that, "He is making more of an effort to succeed in his schoolwork. He is beginning to accept the responsibility for caring for his supplies and for getting to the bus on time. During short periods, Elliott has shown that he can apply himself to schoolwork and make progress. However, these periods are too short and far apart to suggest any consistent gains. Elliott has shown some improvement. Ms. Kimbrough believes he is waking up and she hopes for a big improvement in the next semester."

The report cards from school, which arrived monthly, always indicated something along the lines of, "Elliott has it in him, but we don't know how to get it out of him." Strange how these words were repeated each month. Couldn't someone open Elliott's intricate brain and find out why it was not functioning in a normal fashion? They had so many questions but very few answers!

With Elliott busy at Roosevelt School, my mother's frustrations came out in a different fashion. During the balmy warm days of October, she called a few parents that she had heard about from various sources and invited them to my parent's home to discuss the possibility of a parent association. Several parents attended, but one father in particular, Irving Goldman, who was very concerned about his son's future, became my co-founder of the Cerebral Palsy Parents Association. After several meetings the membership grew too large for my parent's living room to accommodate.

Around the corner from my parent's apartment there was a yellow building that housed the Miami Spiritual and Metaphysical Church's large membership. They opened their doors to the Association and said they could use their facilities at no charge any evening when they did not have prayer meetings or healings. Happy and grateful for the Church's generosity, the group agreed to use the church's facilities on a monthly basis at no charge.

The general consensus of the group was that they were mainly interested in starting a physical therapy clinic. After calling a number of churches, (the location of the metaphysical church wasn't suitable for the clinic) my mother found a sympathetic ear, Minister Lillian, who generously offered use of an empty room in his church's basement. And so the White Temple Methodist Church's basement in downtown Miami became the base for their clinic. The beautiful art deco church with its pink buildings was huge and had many classrooms, which they utilized weekly. A massage table, which was donated by the Polio Foundation, would bring them closer to their goal, but they did not yet have the funds to hire a therapist.

Minister Lillian asked the parents in the group to bring their children to the church for a healing. She also informed them that once a month she did psychic readings. Out of curiosity, my mother went

82

to her on a Sunday to have her give her a reading. To my mother's amazement, Minister Lillian blurted out "Minnie," which was her deceased mother's name, and then proceeded to tell her things about Elliott, although she never met him.

As the group continued to meet monthly, Minister Lillian told them that they could probably attract a therapist to the group by having the newspaper come in and do a story about the organization. Since she was a psychic, Minister Lillian asserted that a story in the newspaper would open the door for them. The *Miami Herald* was their only hope, so my mother called the editor and he sent out a reporter and photographer to my parents home to do the story, complete with pictures. The following Sunday, the *Miami Herald* ran a one-half page feature on the clinic.

"Miami's Forgotten Children Are Going to Get a Break." That was the caption of the story published on April 25, 1948. The article read as follows:

"Parents of children afflicted with cerebral palsy have organized in the hope of rehabilitating some of Miami's 500 youths crippled and distorted by this dreadful malady. Through its long-range program, The Cerebral Palsy Association, Inc. hopes to establish a training school where spastics can be given special attention both medically and intellectually. It wants a separate building to be operated, perhaps in conjunction with The Crippled Children's Society."

"On its immediate agenda is a physical therapy clinic to be held twice weekly, commencing in May, in a room provided by the White Temple Methodist Church. To date, the Cerebral Palsy Association, Inc. has a record of 150 Miami spastics, but based on the national average it is certain that 500 cerebral palsy victims in the greater Miami area under 20 years of age can benefit from the program. The clinic is expected to bring other spastic cases to the association's attention."

"At present, care of spastics is inadequate everywhere. This is not surprising because it is only recently that surveys, classifications, mental testing, and physical diagnosis of spastics have been on a sufficiently large scale to evaluate the problem. With proper attention, thousands of these unfortunate children can be rehabilitated and prepared to lead happier lives. From the Miami Cerebral Palsy Association's efforts, it is hoped that a national foundation might spring."

Along with this publicity was a picture of my mother and Elliott. There was also a story about Gene Boeninger, a law student, and about his fight to become self-sufficient. Today, Gene runs his own printing firm. Gene Boeninger, age 21, and the son of one of the group's members, often came to the meetings when they first organized. The story of Gene's fight to carry on as a normal human being was featured along with my mother and Elliott's publicity.

"I have cerebral palsy," Gene wrote. "More specifically, I am a spastic. I have been this way all my life. My mother first noticed that something was wrong when I couldn't sit up normally at six months of age. Doctors told her that eventually I would overcome most of the difficulties that spastics have to endure. But most important of all, they recognized the fact that I had a normal mentality. That, in it's self, was a milestone because it wasn't so many years ago that spastics were looked upon as being idiots and feeble-minded persons."

"As long as I can remember, I have been under some sort of treatment. Initially, my progress was slow. I could not dress myself, and when I wanted to go to the lavatory somebody always had to help me. In school I was like most other children. Although I was a smart child, it couldn't be seen in most of my work."

"From the start, spelling and reading were my favorite subjects and also my best, but as I grew older, the importance of all aspects of my education became clearer. I gradually came to like school sufficiently to improve my grades and really get down to work. In both grammar and high school there was a separate room for the handicapped where one of two physical therapists were in attendance. We were given exercises to do and some speech correction. I have always been able to feed myself, so my parents haven't had to worry in that direction. But it took eleven years before I could completely dress myself, including buttoning my shirts and tying my shoes. I still have difficulty in closing my shirt collars, however."

"Today I drive my own car and run a printing business in Miami. I will obtain my Bachelor of Business Administration degree in 1949 and law degree from the University of Miami two years later. The very fact that I am a university student makes me realize all the more how lucky I am to be living in this day and age. It wasn't too long ago that victims of cerebral palsy, as I mentioned previously, were automatically assumed to be mentally deficient."

"The grotesque features and drunken gait characteristic of so many spastics helped foster the impression to no end. The biggest difficulty was the fact that spastics could not talk, or if they could, it was often not intelligible except to the immediate family and constant companions."

"Today, doctors are very much aware that spastics possess an average, and in many instances, superior intelligence. In order to bring it to the surface, education should be started at a normal age, and it should not be a standard type, but should fit the child's interests and special needs. If the child becomes disinterested, it is sometimes difficult to for that child to catch up. Therefore, constant monitoring, planning, and adjustments to the educational plan are critical."

"The unfortunate truth is that cerebral palsy is not a rare condition. In fact, it occurs quite regularly in the population at the rate of seven per 100,000 a year in each age group, out of which one dies before the age of development of the brain during pregnancy. In some cases, vitamin deficiencies, glandular disturbances, syphilis, and other systemic diseases during pregnancy are responsible, but most often the cause is the result of some complication during and after birth. Premature and rapid delivery, the use of forceps with heavy pressure, and complications due to the RH factor in the parents' blood, and many other complications are major factors. After birth, convulsions, encephalitis (a type of sleeping sickness), and accidents involving the head may also cause cerebral palsy."

"*Spastic paralysis* is the name of one of the major subdivisions of cerebral palsy. Other types of neuro-muscular crippling conditions included in the general category of cerebral palsy are *athetosis*, or the presence or involuntary motion; *ataxia*, or balance and primary disturbances of coordination; and *rigidity*, or a stiff, lead-like condition of the muscles. These conditions vary considerably, and there is no single type of treatment for cerebral palsy as a whole."

"In treating the various conditions, surgery is not the only answer. Physical therapy, occupational therapy, braces, and drugs are also vital. The most important thing to remember is that the earlier the treatment is begun, the less time bad habits will have to form."

"Four out of six cases are definitely treatable, but two out of the six cases involve feeble-mindedness and require permanent custodial care. The four treatable cases can be divided into three subdivisions. One case will be severely handicapped, homebound, and essentially hopeless from the point of view of physical rehabilitation. Another case will be so mild that any prolonged degree of treatment is unnecessary. Two cases will be moderately handicapped and capable of great improvement. The two cases requiring permanent custodial

86

car are obviously the most severe forms."

As a result of Gene Boeninger's newspaper article, a European physical therapist offered her volunteer services and an orthopedist from Coral Gables agreed to examine the children and prescribe the treatments free of charge. All the furniture and supplies they needed were sent to the church. They were in business!

But then many sad events transpired among the group. One father took his five-year-old daughter's life along with his own by immersing himself and his daughter in a deep canal. Jerry, a young man of 25, who rode his three-wheel bike to my mother's home daily to talk with her in his slurred speech was unable to walk, but she arranged for their doctor to examine him. On his next visit, he informed my mother that the doctor said he was too old to benefit from treatment. Tragically, his body was found in the Miami River the following day. His bike was also found on the banks of the river some distance away.

Immediately my mother was tormented by these tragedies and the fear that the same thing would eventually happen with Elliott. She could see her son's increasing frustration and inability to learn, despite the tests that showed he has a normal mentality.

Most of the group members' children were severely impaired. In fact, only a few could walk. The children sometimes came with their parents to meetings in their mother's arms. Several of the patients suffered from epilepsy and most of them had never attended school because of their handicaps. They never had been exposed to any kind of treatment. By comparison, Elliott was fortunate and blessed.

Charlotte, one of the charter members, told the group about her daughter's tragic birth. Forceps were used and she suffered severe brain damage that left her unable to walk or talk. Although she had been checked by Dr. Winthrop Phelps in Baltimore, there was not much hope for her condition and this affected her parents quite severely. Charlotte's husband died early from a heart attack, but Charlotte continued to work with the group for quite some time.

After several months of the organization's demonstration for the need, they convinced the National Council of Jewish Women to adopt the clinic as a community project. They rented a large storeroom in the southwest section of Miami, and they provided the group with a full-time registered therapist and volunteers to answer the phone and manage the office. They booked all the appointments on a small-scale payment basis, and they raised some monies to cover expenses. First, the patients were examined by the orthopedists who then referred them to the clinic with instructions for treatment. The clinic remained in operation until the United Cerebral Palsy's national organization formed and took over the operation of the existing clinic. It was not long before they built a new, modern facility adjacent to Cedars of Lebanon Hospital near downtown Miami. They were proud to have laid the groundwork.

Although Elliott attended classes at each day at Roosevelt, he was still struggling to acquire an education. He was promoted to the fourth grade socially. His fourth grade teacher, Margaret Jones, reported he was doing better, but that Elliott wasted too much time. "I constantly have to remind Elliott to sit in his seat, his spelling is very poor, and he frequently forgets to do his homework. It's very frustrating, but I just can't seem to get through to him."

Not surprisingly, at the end of fourth grade, Elliott was once again given a social promotion.

Through the efforts of The Crippled Children's Society, a prominent specialist in the field of cerebral palsy was invited down to Miami to examine the children with this affliction, since at the time there was no qualified doctor anywhere in the state of Florida, with the possible exception of Dr. Carlson, who only examined students coming into his boarding school.

Dr. Winthrop Phelps of Baltimore had his own boarding school and clinic. He was often called upon to examine and give his diagnosis throughout the United States. He diagnosed Elliott as a rotary athetoid. This was quite different from Dr. Carlson's report. Dr. Phelp's report read: "He walks with a wide base gait and some unsteadiness. Heel cords adequate length. Hip joints are in normal position in sockets. No limitations of rotation of hip flexion or extension. Abduction fairly strong. External rotators are normal. Internal rotators are apparently weak. Strengthening work should be done in a very internal rotation."

They had just celebrated Elliott's 11th birthday. He was a handsome child, and many friends and relatives joined in on the fun. He had been taking more interest in his schoolwork and one teacher reported that she believed he was "waking up." So much effort had been spent trying to find the key to motivate him, so this was very welcome news. New hope rose within my mother. And then one day Elliott came home from school and said: "Here, mother, take my crutches and put them away. I won't need them anymore."

"Our son is walking, our son is walking alone," my mother shouted to my father when he arrived home from work. "Look, Eddie, I put his crutches in the garage." Even though he was tired from a hard day at the drugstore, my father danced around the living room with my mother. They both kissed Elliott and gave him lots of hugs for his decision, his courage, and his ability to walk alone.

When school opened in the fall, the handicapped children were placed under the medical and orthopedic care of The Crippled Children's Society. This time Dr. Harriett Gillette, a cerebral palsy specialist from Atlanta, was the attending physician. My mother was invited to observe the examination. Her diagnosis was a mixture of rotary athetoid and ataxia spastic. Physical therapy was recommended and high-laced shoes were prescribed. In occupational therapy, Elliott had to strive for dexterity. Speech therapy was also prescribed.

Some friends of my parents had two children, one normal and one with cerebral palsy. We were invited to their home for birthday cake to celebrate when their normal child became one year old. Their older daughter was sitting in a wheelchair, unable to speak, but mentally alert. We noted the happiness on the faces of this mother and father and felt the great love radiating from all the members of the family for the healthy little toddler. My mother could think of nothing except the warmth she felt in their home. On the way home, my parents decided it was time to add to their family. It was the birthday party that made up my mother's mind.

The years of 1949 and 1950 brought two major blessings. Elliott was walking on his own, and my parents learned that they had a baby due in October 1950. The house was bursting with excitement. There was so much to do and think about.

Because of my mother's strong desire to help disabled children, she volunteered her services with The Crippled Children's Society. They welcomed her with open arms, for they knew her background with cerebral palsy. She was immediately made an honorary board member and put in charge of the "Easter Lily Day" collection. My mother's first assignment was to take Elliott to see Sophie Tucker, a popular nightclub singer who was booked at a local club. She was to interview Ms. Tucker and accept her donation in the canister. The *Miami Herald* took a picture, which appeared in the paper the following day.

Then came an opportunity for my father to open a small pharmacy in a medical building and he quickly jumped at the chance. The emotional challenge of having another business of his own was just the thing he needed to stimulate his interest in life again. My mother's friendship with the president of the National Council of Jewish Women opened the door for my parents. Her husband was a medical doctor who had just built a clinic near the *Miami Herald*, and he was looking for a pharmacist to open the store in the space reserved for that purpose. My father opened his latest business with enthusiasm and it had the promise of becoming a profitable business. He only had to keep the doctor's hours, which were a reasonable five and a half days per week.

After Dr. Gillette examined Elliott again, she reported that his emotional problems were now becoming more pronounced as he was aging. He was experiencing severe temper tantrums. She recommended a new school in Alabama and my parents considered it for the future. They were both tormented by the report and started to think that Elliott might have some level of retardation. They had to look toward and perhaps find some permanent home for Elliott. My mother's search for a diagnosis and treatment of Elliott's condition was over at last. Now they knew what they were facing. Elliott had been treated by the best doctors in the country. My mother's refusal to accept the hopelessness, which doctors had tried to force upon her had now, to a great degree, been rewarded. Elliott could talk, he could walk, and he was in a school program. Not all his physical or educational problems were solved, but most of them were out of my mother's hands.

The following report by Dr. Seymour Blumenthal, a psychologist, was sent to my parents after his evaluation:

"On the Revised Stanford-Binet, Form L, Elliott attains a mental age of 8-4, and an IQ of 81, indicating dull-normal intelligence. His range of testing is from year Level VII through year Level X. His vocabulary development, as indicated by his ability to define words, is at the ten-year level of expectancy. His judgment and reasoning abilities are variable and, on the whole, quite immature. However, there are indications that there is a basically better range of ability in these areas. Retention is likewise variable with the concomitant of poor mental control as well as evidence of difficulty in learning for this reason."

"A series of performance tests were administered to this boy, but as was already known, Elliott's severe handicap is the use of his hands and fingers which do not permit for any comparison with known standards. On the basis of a qualitative evaluation of his functioning--partially out of the interference due to muscular difficulties--the boy indicates that his range of ability is of approximate range."

"In general, his development in the basic school skills of reading and arithmetic are not too well established. He has some simple word recognition, but it is not adequate for satisfactory comprehension in text materials; his ability along arithmetical lines is severely retarded."

"It is this examiner's impression that the present test results are not at all representative of his basic mental abilities. To a large extent, the present test results are a reflection of very poor habits, which have been instituted in his study and general overall adjustment so that he does not at all make use of what appears to be at least average mental ability status. In general, he will not extend himself to give adequate impression of his basic mental ability structure. To a large extent, much of the present difficulty in adjustment, as well as in ineffective use of his basic mental abilities, must be attributed to over-protection and a lack of stimulation and motivation, which would tend to make him more effective. The parents, while meaning well, have done very little to install a plan of discipline which would make him a more effective child in line with his basic mental abilities. At the present time, the boy is infantile, demanding, and utilizes every avenue to control his parents and therefore avoids accepting responsibility which he can apparently handle. This dependence, and the advantage that he takes of his parents, will subsequently set a behavior pattern which will be most difficult to control and which, in general, will tend for maladjustment. Effective management as well as a specific plan of discipline for the child is of paramount importance."

"Recommendations: This is not a problem of intellective retardation, but rather interference in the use of his approximate average mental abilities due to personality problems which have been more or less conditioned by over-protection of the parents. He is, therefore, not effectively using his basic abilities and is presenting a very inadequate picture of them. His parents were counseled to formulate a plan which would be in line with the boy's abilities and wherein they would be able to maintain gradually increasing programs, which make optimal use of his basic abilities for adjustment. From the school point of view, the boy is retarded in the basic school skills, but this likewise is a reflection of this boy's unwillingness to extend his self, which stems initially from home. If both the parents and school can coordinate their activities for an adequate plan of discipline for this child, a more effective adjustment should be noted. Remedial education should be instituted at the earliest opportunity."

My parents never discussed their feelings about Elliott. It was like they were in a silent conspiracy not to speak out loud about how Elliott's problems affected them, as if the result of voicing their emotions would somehow make things worse. My father had suffered silently, often leaving the major action to my mother. Did he refuse to accept the facts of Elliott's world of reality? He was a kind and loyal husband, but he found it difficult to bare his soul.
Dr. Blumenthal's report gave my parents further insight into Elliott's condition and his possible future education. Apparently, Dr. Carlson had overestimated Elliott's capabilities, perhaps because he was much younger then and more difficult to analyze.

Chapter 6
My Birth

The days passed quickly during my mother's nine months of pregnancy. She looked forward to the delivery of a normal baby, as well as getting back to her original size eight dress.

My mother was under special care of Dr. Leon Greene, their medical gynecologist friend who rented space in the physician's building where my father ran his pharmacy. He assured my mother that everything was normal and not to be concerned; he would take care of her just like he would his own daughter. During her last examination, Dr. Gillette had recommended a new summer camp for Elliott in the hills of North Carolina. She thought Elliott would benefit greatly from the camp. My mother kept busy by labeling his camp clothes and by preparing the layette for their expected newborn.

Elliott left for camp in June for two months. He flew alone but was monitored by the flight attendant and met by Travelers Aid to make sure he boarded the right bus for camp. The local newspaper took pictures and he was photographed getting off the plane in Blowing Rock. He was a celebrity!

Elliott had a wonderful experience at Camp Sky Ranch, which had just opened that summer for handicapped children. He had many stories to tell and took a lot of pictures with the Brownie camera, which my parents bought for him because it was relatively easy to use. Nonetheless, many of his pictures were actually taken by others, once he had composed the shot.

September was a bustling time. My parents had to purchase a crib, a dressing table, and chest of drawers. It was going to be a tight fit for the small bedroom they had available, but they would manage until they had the money to buy a larger home. All the arrangements were made with Sarah to stay with Elliott while my mother was in the hospital. She would also prepare the breakfast and dinner meals during that time.

Elliott was so excited about having a sister or brother in the family. He had been the only child for almost twelve years. My mother had often thought about having another child, but did not think she could cope with both and do them equal justice. Elliott needed special time for his educational and emotional needs.

Elliott's twelfth birthday was in September. Family members came over to celebrate with cake and ice cream and they brought some new clothes for Elliott, too. By now they knew that the shirts Elliott wore must be pull-on's and that his pants had to have an elastic waist. The time for my mother's delivery was getting closer, her stomach protruding as if it housed an over-inflated basketball. She sensed that this child would be a girl, although a powerful kicker. There was a lot more activity than with Elliott when she had carried him. He had kicked very little and was rather light. For the first time, my mother came to realize that whatever was wrong with Elliott had begun while she was carrying him, and that the problems were only worsened by the difficult nature of his delivery with Dr. Craft.

My mother awoke that night to pitch darkness and was immediately alert. What was it that had aroused her so quickly? Then she felt the cramp-like pain low in her back. The time had come! She wanted to wake my father but decided to wait a little while. It might be a long time and my father would need all the rest he could get.

My mother's mind was spinning. The pregnancy had been normal; she had not experienced any nausea beyond what was normal for any woman during the first three months. But as she lay in bed thinking of what this day might bring, she knew she was terribly afraid of the final outcome. Could there be something wrong with her that made it impossible for her to give birth to a normal child? Would the birth process be handed skillfully? With these thoughts clouding

95

her mind, she was filled with increasing fear at the approach of her child's birth. My mother was terrified that she would have to relive the unspeakable tragedy of Elliott's entrance into the world.

My mother's body stiffened. She wanted to shout, "Damn that doctor in Pennsylvania!" It suddenly became clear that her anger toward Dr. Craft had become deep and strong. She had kept her anger deep inside all those years, voicing only a cool but objective analysis of Elliott's birth. She had tried many times to find out what had gone wrong, but without success. She felt chills run up my spine as the pain came again. "God," She prayed. "Take away my rage! Help me to be reasonable. I know I am desperately afraid. Oh please, God, don't let it happen again, not again!"

She woke my father, dressed, and called Sarah to come and stay with Elliott. Then they were on their way to the hospital.

After the interminable storm passed, a nurse with a beaming smile placed into my mother's arms the most beautiful baby girl she had ever seen. I was a tiny, 6 ½ pound child, they named me Marlene. I had arrived at 11:00 A.M. My mother could not believe that this porcelain doll with brushed up curls around the back of her head and a snookie roll of hair on the top was her baby. She thought they had made a mistake in the nursery, but the tiny row of plastic beds the size of a quarter said "Weiss." There was no error. I was their baby girl.

My mother fell into a light sleep. Later she was awakened by a kiss on her forehead. My father stood by her side with a big grin on his face, holding a dozen dark red roses in one hand and a package under his arm. "We're very lucky," he said smiling. Even if he had tried, there was no way he could have hidden the excitement, joy, and relief on his face and in his eyes.

"Eddie, this is the first time you have ever given me roses except for my birthday. And that package, you old dear, what have you brought me?"

He stood silently as my mother carefully untied the precious ribbon on the package. In the box was an exquisite blue nightgown. Their hands touched and, still in silence, their eyes met for a long moment.

A little later my father said, "For 12 years, Rose, you have dedicated your life to Elliott. I'm sure your hope and courage have played a large role in seeing Elliott walk. And you have received the reward of his words, his speech. But what will happen now? Have you thought about what this new baby will do to our lives, especially Elliott's?"

"Well, you know I haven't been a pampering mother, have I?"

"No."

"Don't worry about where Marlene will fit into this picture. I've already been dreaming what it will be like to raise a normal child. I'll dedicate my efforts to giving her a normal, happy life just as ardently as I have worked for Elliott. I'll make room in my life for both of them. Marlene must learn very early to respect and accept her handicapped brother."

Dr. Greene came into my mother's room. "Congratulations on your beautiful, healthy, normal daughter." Dr. Greene went on to explain that he had done just a little cutting (an episiotomy) just to make sure everything would be fine. "She's also been examined by the pediatrician and he's given us a glowing report." Dr. Greene sat with my mother for a while and explained to her why she should not have had any previous problem delivering a normal baby. Then, she thought, it must have been something Dr. Craft had done wrong which had caused Elliott's brain damage. But then again, she had to accept that she would never truly know what went wrong with her boy.

Each time she walked to the nursery to admire her baby, my mother noticed I was not in my crib but in the lap of the nurse while she was doing her charts. Stretched out on her stomach with the nurse patting me on the back, I went to sleep. My mother knocked on the window to get the nurse's attention. She wanted to know why her baby wasn't in her bed. The nurse smiled at her and said, "Because she is the cutest one here, the pride of the nursery and a very good baby. She hardly ever cries."

To that, my mother replied, "OK, but don't spoil her too much."

At the end of the week, it was time to leave the hospital and go home. Uncle Julius and Aunt Tillie arrived shortly before lunch to escort my parents home. Aunt Tillie held me tightly, for this baby was going to be her new love. Their small home was bursting at the seams. Sarah had decorated the living room with a big "Welcome" sign and had tied colorful balloons all over the room. It was a Saturday and Elliott was home too. A beautiful lunch was on the table and my mother felt like a queen for a day. Sarah, who now had a nurse's degree, had taken three weeks off from her job to care for me. It was a wonderful gesture, for she was always in demand, but her and my mother's friendship over the past twelve years had been steadfast. Since my mother brought her to Florida, despite the many changes in their lives, she had always remained grateful.

I had the usual three-month colic. My parents took turns at night walking me or pushing my carriage back and forth until I went back to sleep. Watching the growth of a normal child was a new experience for them. I did everything according to the book. I sat up at six months old and danced my version of the "hula" to Arthur Godfrey's guitar music, Hawaiian style. I played with my rattles and toys without any lessons or teachers. Everything came automatically. My mother told everyone there wasn't anything more interesting in this world than watching the development of a normal child. I was such a contrast to Elliott, and my mother didn't want to miss a moment of this pleasure. I had my periodical examinations and immunizations at due times. At the age of one, I walked, could say "mama" and "dada," and even "bubba" for my brother. I loved to play with all my toys and even had a little girl to play with in the neighborhood.

That spring, Elliott completed his grades on a social level at Roosevelt and was transferred to the Ada Merritt Junior High School, where he was placed on a social level rather than on an academic level. Ada Merritt provided bus service and had special classrooms for the handicapped youngsters, as well as classes for mainstream students. It was at that point in his life when Elliott showed a renewed interest in carpentry. Ada Merritt did not use the report card system, but instead issued progress reports on a social scale. The classes were small and students graduated at 18 years of age. In fact, Elliott remained there until he turned 18, at which point he was awarded a social diploma. Today this is known as "aging out of the system."

Not knowing quite what to do with Elliott at that point, my parents weighed the situation very carefully and decided to follow Dr. Gillette's advice to try the Charlanne School in Birmingham, Alabama. It was a new boarding school for the handicapped. Since it was a private school, this would mean smaller classes and more time per student. They were willing to take this last educational chance to see if Elliott would benefit. Perhaps some vocation would interest Elliott so that he could have a productive future. Therapy would also be included, so they hoped they would continue helping him with his walking, speech, and muscle coordination. In September of 1956, Elliott flew to Birmingham to register for Charlanne's fall and spring semesters.

My parents kept in close touch with Elliott and received regular reports. The school informed my parents that his academic work was improving. He was doing a little better in reading, and geography and science were of great interest to him. He was doing fourth-grade work in these two subjects and eagerly hunted for science stories in

99

his *Weekly Reader*. His language comprehension was also on the fourth-grade level, and he seemed to understand sentence construction, correct usage of words, letter writing, and story telling.

Elliott's teachers at Charlanne believed he could make more rapid progress, but only if he would exert himself. They all agreed that he still needed encouragement if he was to achieve a higher level of independence, and that he needed coaching in initiative in high academic work and everyday activities.

Prior to Christmas vacation, Elliott was given the Stanford-Binet Intelligence Test and the results indicated he was normal mentally. It seemed the major cause of his problems was that he was a typical teenager who wasn't eager to apply himself. How my mother wanted to believe them! If the key to his learning difficulties could be found, then Elliott might have a profession he could pursue, despite his physical handicaps. Part of my mother continued to hope, but serious doubts continued to linger in her mind.

The progress report at the end of May seemed to be a bit more encouraging. "Elliott is reading in the new *If I Were Going* reader, which is a hard third- level reader. He interprets the contents of the stories with a great deal of exactness when the stories are read orally, but he is unable to give a very clear interpretation when the story has been read silently. Elliott enjoys Word Drill period, as he does nicely with the sounds of letters and the pronouncing of new words, and most of the time he interprets the correct meaning of the new words."

"Elliott seems to understand sentence construction, correct usage of words, letter writing, and story telling. Elliott has begun spelling on the fifth grade level, but this progress requires more time than he wishes to give; therefore, he is not too happy about his advancement in spelling. He has a very good conception of the use of the dictionary, arranging words in alphabetical order, and doing diction work. Elliott works at a very slow rate of speed when working independently."

"Elliott moved along faster in fourth grade arithmetic when he was adding and subtracting, but when he reached multiplication and division he made very slow progress. Elliott moves very slowly when working independently in arithmetic."

"The typewriter has been a joy to Elliott and a great help, too. He has shown a steady improvement in his use of the typewriter. He tried very hard to use the correct finger on the correct key and to learn the entire use of the typewriter. His typewriter has been a great help to him in his classroom studies. He has used it very successfully for work in geography, spelling, and language."

"We believe that Elliott could make more rapid progress with greater effort because he seems capable of better work than he does; however, Elliott does better and faster work when under complete supervision. However, independently he seems to progress at a slow rate of speed and lacks concentration. Without close supervision, he goes on to other activities instead of concentrating on the assigned work."

"He seems to enjoy collecting articles and is very appreciative of what is given to him, but he lacks determined effort to do things for himself at times. He seems to enjoy annoying other people and children younger than himself, but he will apologize when corrected. Efforts should be continued to help Elliott grow to become more independent in his work habits. We believe he has improved considerably this school year and has "grown up" to a great extent, but, of course, he still needs encouragement to develop more independence and more initiative in his work and in his everyday activities."

Chapter 7
Mom's Dedication to My Life

Dry-wood termites had invaded my parent's duplex, so they had the place tented, but it only helped temporarily because the persistent little bugs returned again in the spring. Once again, it was time to look for a new, larger, home where they would be more comfortable.

Soon we found a newly constructed home on Southwest 18th Avenue, which had been sitting vacant six months after its completion.

"It's a big, beautiful home," my father said after he'd first seen the house, located in a neighborhood where he'd delivered some prescriptions. "Here's the number for the builder. Call them and arrange for us to see the inside." My mother followed father's suggestion, and immediately she fell in love with the place. Within minutes she could visualize how the rooms would look furnished. The builder, Mr. Stevens, was anxious to sell the house, so he agreed to take my parents duplexes in trade, with the balance in cash. They were ecstatic. They now had a new, large, permanent home, a new pharmacy, and a beautiful, normal daughter. They were also looking for peaceful solutions for Elliott's future. Indeed, they were beginning to feel very lucky.

My mother shopped for furniture for the three bedrooms, and after explaining the various pieces to my father he reluctantly nodded his head in approval. Within a few days my mother had found a French provincial bedroom set for my room and a white Italian provincial suite for her and my father's bedroom. For Elliott's room my mother purchased a single bed, bookcases, a desk for his typewriter, and a chest of drawers, all suitable for a typical teenage boy's room. They also bought a new table and chairs for the kitchen and a rattan set for the screen-enclosed front porch. To save some money, they decided that new furnishings for the living and dining rooms could wait until later, although they did buy a large new television set.

They took time selecting the artwork for their new home. They would shop on Saturdays after my father came home from the store. In addition to its annual art show, Coconut Grove, an area located at the southern end of Miami overlooking Biscayne Bay, was home to many beautiful galleries that they enjoyed shopping in.

Then Elliott, who was now twenty years old, came home again after his two-year tenure at Charlanne. My parents purchased an adult three-wheel bicycle for him so he could ride around and meet their neighbors. Unfortunately, despite their son's friendly efforts to meet new people, the neighbors just weren't receptive to Elliott. They just wished that Elliott could have found at least one young man in his age group to talk to or go places with. Just one friend would have made such a difference in his life. In this beautiful community that they loved so much, the same dark cloud began to appear on the horizon each beautiful day. While my mother's heart filled with joy for me, it ached for Elliott. Despite his disappointing efforts to make new friends, Elliott always remained upbeat and friendly and optimistic that he would eventually make new friends.

One day our neighbors informed me that a new family had purchased the white three-bedroom house across the street. The family consisted of three daughters, a teenager, a two-year-old, and a three-month-old baby. Until now, there were no young children who lived in the immediate area.

A few days after our new neighbors moved in, my mother had her first encounter with Maxine, their two-year-old daughter. She wheeled me over to their house after one of our afternoon strolls. As we entered the front porch, Maxine was staring through the screen door.   As soon as my mother said "Hello," she heard the quick response, "Can I come over to your house to play?" My mother quickly answered, "Yes, we would love to have you."

My newfound friendship with Maxine was cemented quickly and we became fast friends. Jean, Maxine's mother, was also very friendly. My mother and her quickly learned that they shared a common bond; Jean's sister had been born with cerebral palsy. Jean worked side by side with her husband, Morris, at a supermarket in Miami, so her and my mother's time together was limited. However, they did spend Wednesdays together with their girls. They would go to the beach, go toy shopping, or attend social activities that their girls were involved in.

Meanwhile, Elliott's daily bicycle rides continued to be more important to him because they gave him a sense of freedom, but the neighbors continued to shut their doors on him. As a result, Elliott began riding his three-wheeler down to Coral Way, where he met and visited some of the local merchants he'd met before his two years at Charlanne; some of the merchants were receptive to him, but others, of course, were not.

During this time, my parents had a little more money at their disposal than they had previously. They enjoyed spending their Saturday afternoons with their two children, at various department stores around town, shopping for their clothing and other necessities. My mother still had not learned to drive (that would come some years later) so in order to get around, she had to depend on my father, which was difficult, because he was spending so much of his time working. Something my parents enjoyed immensely were frequent dinners at the Biscayne Cafeteria on Miracle Mile in Coral Gables, where they dined as often as two or three times a week.

In addition to immediate family, more of my father's relatives from up north were migrating to Florida and settling in. They enjoyed the togetherness that this allowed and everyone got together whenever possible.

During this time, my mother was a member of the National Council of Jewish Women. She was faithful to the group because of the good fortune that came to my parents as a result of her acquaintance with one of the members, Sylvia Levin. Sylvia's husband was a well-established ophthalmologist in the Physician's Building on North Bayshore Drive. It was Dr. Levin who put my father in touch with the landlords of the building after suggesting that this would be a smart place for him to open his new business. Although my father wouldn't get much walk-in traffic in such a store, it was clear that he would always be busy, filling prescriptions for patients seeing doctors in the building. Fortunately, he took Dr. Levin's advice, and for about ten years he ran this successful pharmacy until he became too ill to continue working, at which point he sold off the inventory and shut the doors.

As a board member of the National Council of Jewish Women, my mother suggested that the group collect educational toys for the pre-school kindergarten children in Israel at Hanukkah time. This project was named "Ship a Box," and after much consideration, my mother's suggestion was accepted and implemented on a national level.

While Elliott attended a two-week summer camp, the rest of the family went to a summer resort nearby in Asheville, North Carolina. My father decided to go to Duke University Medical Center to see if they could diagnose the burning sensation he had been experiencing in his tongue. As it turned out, the ensuing report was that he had become diabetic. This news came as a shock at first, but then my parents finally accepted it as something else they would have to live with. My father's mother had also developed diabetes, so this was apparently a genetic misfortune and should not have come as

105

much of a surprise.

Another health problem also presented itself at about the same time. I presented the first evidence of asthma. My first asthma attack was brought on after sleeping on a feather pillow one night. For a frightened moment, it seemed to my parents that I might be less than healthy. Fortunately, however, my asthma has never been much of a hindrance. I was an active child, and as an adult I continue to be an energetic woman.

As I was growing up, my mother constantly marveled at the easiness of my growth and maturity. As a student in school, I always understood everything that was being taught. I smiled whenever anyone spoke to me and my mother always marvelled at my precise coordination. As a child, I was full of love and laughter and every day I brightened the household with my countenance.

One day my mother entered the living room and found my father lying on the sofa with the evening paper discarded on the stool beside him. He seemed not to notice her, but then he said quietly, "Sit down, Rose. It's time we took a good look at where we are with Elliott. He has been in so many schools—very good schools— Charlanne being one of them."

"Eddie," my mother said to him. "What are you getting at?"

"I'm just pointing out the reality: Elliott is 21 years old now and he's still functioning on a third grade level. What does that tell us, Rose? Let's be truly honest with each other about this for once. Of course we both want so much to believe that the magic key will be found to change things, but how far are we supposed to take this fantasy that he's going to suddenly get well? Where else is there to turn? All these years I've watched you devote your energy to searching, working, and studying how to help Elliott. You've had so little of your own life. As long as your efforts and the special schools were helping him, I had no problem, but I've begun to wonder how

106

much of this has been worth it. I just can't stand to see Elliott pushed anymore. I don't say a lot, Rose and you know I've gone along with you, even though it meant keeping us drained financially. But let's face it. Deep down you know as well as I that although no authority has had the courage to tell us, we must accept--we must face the truth that--"

Eddie was struggling to say it but kept avoiding the word. I finally interrupted him by finishing his statement. "Elliott is retarded."

"Yes, that's right, Rose. I'm sorry, but Elliott is retarded."

Both of us were quiet for a long moment, letting the fact take shape.

"Eddie, it truly seems to me now that all the testing, the reports, and the remarks uttered by the string of professionals we've consulted are a shapeless mass of meaningless words. No one—not one—has provided us with a solution. For a long time I've been studying the school reports and I, too, have been wondering how long we can further torture our poor brain-damaged son in order to give him an education. Besides, how much longer can we spend so much money on experiment after experiment, because that's just what it has been—experimenting. It isn't right. It's not fair to push Elliott, and it isn't fair to us. We better start getting used to the truth we have skirted for so long. At least it will help us relax with him better. You're right, Eddie, I'm not going to push so hard any more."

Relief and pain flooded my mother. Now they both knew what the situation was and they could attempt to deal with it.

Elliott had demonstrated that he knew his basic mathematical processes quite well, he could read with understanding, but he disliked writing. His only true interest in school had been working with tools in the wood shop. Ironically, he did get a thrill from being able to do his spelling well, but his refusal to write rendered this capability somewhat meaningless.

107

Emotionally, Elliott was still trying hard to exert control over his self. He was conscious that a lack of control repelled people rather than attracted them. This disturbed Elliott because his greatest desire was to have friends and be appreciated. To my parent's frustration, he showed no interest in anything academic or vocational. He needed very much to be more relaxed so that his speech could be improved. If only Elliott could concentrate on something of vital interest to him, it would have given him a greater sense confidence. It was so important for Elliott's emotional survival for him to be able to do something well.

A new sheltered workshop had opened up near the house and Elliott was permitted to try working with them for one week. The facility offered jobs for people with assorted physical and mental handicaps. Unfortunately, Elliott's inability to concentrate on the work assigned to him caused the director to dismiss Elliott.

My parents had never discussed institutional care for Elliott, but the idea was creeping into mind. Nonetheless, my mother tried my best to fight these thoughts. "Elliott is still young," She would often say to herself. "Perhaps we should wait awhile and see what the future will bring."

She had never visited an institution for either mentally or physically retarded patients. Such state-operated residences held the reputation of being cold, hostile places. She could only visualize old, large cement block buildings housing 100 people huddled into crowded dormitories with only a small recreation room for television or games. In her mind, she was envisioning a facility not much different from a prison, a thought that broke her heart, because Elliott is the kindest, most peaceful man you could ever hope to meet.

After visiting Farm Colony, a state institution for the retarded in Gainesville, my parents were convinced that their fears were unjustified. My mother knew Elliott would be much happier with other young men his own age. The buildings of the institution were old but well kept. The residential areas were immaculate and clients were dressed in clean, suitable clothing. The staff was warm and receptive and gave my parents an excellent tour. They had expected the worst, so they were greatly relieved and more relaxed than they had been for a long, long time. Knowing the day would come soon, dreading it, and remembering stories about state institutions, a great tension had built up inside of them. The time had come to place the application.

It was a hot summer day when my mother took the bus to downtown Miami. As was often the case in those years, my father didn't feel well enough to get dressed and drive. As you can imagine, the situation was excruciating for my mother. Her only prior experience at the courthouse was when she had gone there to apply for Homestead Exemption on their homes. This time the trip was different: she was committing Elliott to the State of Florida.

Thoughts filled her mind. Primarily she kept wondering if Elliott would remain in Gainesville forever? There were no answers. She nervously waited for her turn to see the judge. Finally, she was ushered into his chambers. The judge was an elderly man, kind and compassionate. He showed his sympathy with his soft-spoken words and his gentle actions. He touched her shoulder and explained that it would take approximately two years for Elliott to be accepted into the program, as the waiting list was very long and they had only a few vacancies. He said openings were usually available when a resident died. Furthermore, he said that parents never took their children out once they were admitted to the facility.

To some extent, Farm Colony, which was later renamed Sunland, was a dumping ground for all sorts of defective, deformed, brain-damaged, handicapped people, from infants to the elderly. Each cottage housed 40 people, according to their age and intelligence bracket, and this is where they lived, worked, and played together.

My mother's mind was reeling as she bid the judge goodbye and thanked him for being so kind. On the bus ride home, she continued to weigh the situation. Even though it was hard to think about the decision they had made, it seemed that Farm Colony could do more for Elliott than they could at home. Besides the school and workshop, Farm Colony had a lot of planned recreational activities. "How fortunate," she thought, "that parents with normal children do not have to make these kinds of decisions." She thought about the life my father and her had planned to live and how things had turned out. Were they being punished for something they had done wrong? Why had this happened to them? To Elliott?

While all of this was going on, I was in the process of growing up. Each morning my mother would walk Maxine and I to Coral Way Elementary School, the same school that had refused admission to Elliott. Then, for safety reasons--the neighborhood had changed since we'd first moved in—my mother would go back to the school and walk us home. It was so comforting for my mother to see her daughter learning so much so fast. My report cards were all complimentary— such a contrast to Elliott's reports.

Despite my parent's earlier disappointment with that school, they found Coral Way Elementary to be a very active school with an outstanding principal and an active PTA. My teacher believed in keeping the students involved in many of the extra-curricular events offered at the school including drama, art, and music. To keep astride with my interests, my mother became a PTA member and attended all the meetings. My mother didn't want to miss out on anything that I was involved with. My normal maturity, which most mothers took for granted in their children, was a new world for her and she didn't want to miss a moment of it.

She even worked in the cafeteria at lunchtime passing out the cartons of milk and she also became chairman of many committees just to keep abreast of ongoing programs. I loved school and was an excellent student.

At this point, my parents didn't know how long they would have to wait for Elliott to be accepted into Farm Colony. He would pass these days following his routine. In the mornings and afternoons he would ride his bike to Coral Way to visit his merchant friends. Along the way, he would often stop and speak with the garbage men, gardeners, the mailman, the milkman, and anyone else who would pay him some attention. Then he would visit his friend Bill, who ran a small hardware store on Coral Way and Southwest 17th Avenue. Bill sold plants and seeds of all kinds. He was a compassionate man and a good listener. Then Elliott would visit Jack to inspect his latest project. Then by dinnertime, Elliott would head home. Despite these positive contacts, this was a lonesome and uneventful time for Elliott. The need for recreation and a workshop was a dire necessity in our community, but there wasn't anyone with the money and the interest to create such a facility.

Not surprisingly, I kept begging for a sibling, even a cat or dog, to keep me company. Since having another baby was out of the question, we settled for a white Persian cat who we named Snowy. However, Snowy's time with us was short lived because of my terrible allergies. Then Collette, our new white poodle, took Snowy's place. She became my dog and followed me everywhere. The following spring Collette gave birth to four adorable puppies, which we gave to friends.

Then one spring afternoon the long-awaited letter arrived from the State of Florida. They now had room for Elliott and would accept him at Farm Colony in Gainesville. Once again, my mother was in a state of emotional turmoil. Throughout that day, she tormented my father with a barrage of questions: "Are we doing the right thing? Is this really best for Elliott? How can we part with him? What will our lives be like without him? How will he survive without us? Eddie, are we being selfish? Are we making the right choice? Is this best for Elliott?"

It had been one thing to make the application, but it was another to actually be faced with the separation. My parents spent a rather restless, sleepless night as they lived through the decision-making process one more time. Finally, they began thinking rational again as they had before the letter arrived. The storm had passed. Elliott was headed for Gainesville, some 335 miles to the north of Miami.

"We will visit Elliott as often as possible and we'll bring him home for vacations and holidays," my father said reassuringly. "Rose, we've given him the best education possible and the best medical care available. Now all we can do is hope he'll learn a trade to carry him through and that he will be happy."

The emotional impact of parting struck my mother so hard that she knew she could not be the one to take him to Farm Colony. Fortunately, they learned that private-car service was available and that other young adults were leaving on the same day.

While taping Elliott's name on his clothes, my mother explained to him that he would be going to a new school in Gainesville where he would have a workshop in which he could learn to make things. She told Elliott he would make new friends and assured him that she would visit him often and that he would visit on holidays.

Morning came warm and clear and my mother faced the family peacefully and efficiently, making sure Elliott's clothes were ready and his suitcase was packed. We all walked Elliott to the waiting car to join the other children and said goodbye without putting him through the emotional storm my parents faced. He waved contentedly through the side window and then he was gone.

Together, my parents slowly walked back into the house. My mother told her self that she had learned many times it is not good to brood, and once a decision is made, acceptance and involvement in new things is best. With this in mind, she became even busier with my school activities.

But first there was that first evening without Elliott. This, of course, was a terribly sad time for my parents. My mother tried to keep her spirits up, but it was difficult. Tears kept running down her face and I kept asking, "What is wrong, Mommy?" As my mother wiped her eyes, all she could say was, "I am going to miss Elliott very much." She turned away from me as she said, "You will understand this better as you get older." Her only consolation was that she felt confident that Elliott would make friends, which had been impossible in our neighborhood. The past years had been so emotional and time consuming; my parent's thought perhaps now was a time for peace and bliss with me, their daughter. I would bring joy and laughter into their lives. The tide would be changing, the storm would be over, and the sun would be shining for all of us.

In fact, the next few years were often joyous for us. Everything seemed special, even the simple act of walking with my friends and I while we skipped along. My mother felt almost as if it were a dream. How great it was to see that not only could I speak well and walk with grace and ease, but I could also run, skip, hop, and jump!

When the time arrived for me to join the Girl Scouts, my mother took the standard training course to become a Brownie Girl Scout leader, given by the Girl Scout Council of Dade County. Eighteen eight-year-old girls from two nearby schools joined the group, Troop #115. Two assistant leaders helped my mother. Volunteer mothers and three other women on the committee also assisted me in various duties.

Our many planned activities included the "young people's concert and a Halloween party for which the girls made their own paper costumes and went to Camp Mahachee for a nature hike and picnic. This was a combined trip with another Brownie troop. We stuffed dolls for patients at Farm Colony, enjoyed a nature trip to Matheson Hammock, gathered plants to start a terrarium, and we visited the Crandon Park Zoo. We also toured the local museums and the Fairchild Tropical Gardens, saw a taping of the *Jim Dooly Show*, and had a Mother's Day Tea. We wrote and presented a one-act play entitled, "The Mothers, They Forgot." Other times we had dinners at Shorty's Barbecue or went on hayrides at the Circle B Ranch in Davie. Our family picnic at Crandon Park and a trip to the *Miami Herald* circulation and printing departments culminated our year's events.

Our services to the community were many. Part of each meeting was spent stuffing dolls and animals, making scrap books, and preparing Christmas gifts which were all sent to the Farm Colony in Gainesville, the Mental Health Society, United Cerebral Palsy of Miami, and the Girl Scout Council of Dade County.

Our Brownies were invested again to the intermediate level and became Girl Scouts. But on our final day, we announced that we were no longer interested in becoming Girl Scouts. Our interests had changed and we were more interested in boys. And that ended my mother's Girl Scout career. She was sad, but she thanked everyone anyway. At least we had three years of good citizenship, and learned how to be compassionate for those less fortunate. We gained the love and satisfaction of giving to others, learned about nature, and became better persons. Our Brownie vows were fulfilled and my mother felt gratified that she had contributed to our young lives.

Meanwhile, in the spring of 1962, Sunland Training Center in Fort Myers opened its doors. At the same time, Farm Colony's name was changed to Sunland Training Center. This meant Elliott could be transferred to Fort Myers. This translated into a shorter trip than we'd been making, as Fort Myers was so much closer than Gainesville was. This way, we could visit Elliott once a month. In fact, we visited Elliott the first Saturday after he was transferred to Fort Myers. The newly painted cottages and roofs sparkled like snow in the sun. The grounds resembled a college campus.

Elliott gave us a grand tour, but we were disappointed to find that there was no air conditioning in the cottages. The sleeping quarters had large fans, but the day room, where the residents ate and watched television, was extremely hot. There wasn't a breath of cool air during the long summer days. My mother's first thought was that we had to get those cottages cooled.

Naturally she got involved in the formation of the Sunland Parents Association and they agreed that their first project was to raise money for air conditioners. As the first president of the association, my mother decided that they would create a trading stamp fund raising project to raise the necessary money. It took about two years to complete this project, but she'll always be proud of their successful efforts.

As Elliott matured, his desire to work increased. Although his teachers tried to encourage him with various rehabilitation programs, it was difficult for him to feel fulfilled by any of them. Since he rode a large tricycle, Elliott was anxious to do some kind of work in which he could use his bike. He was allowed to deliver messages from one area to another. Elliott was delighted. He was outdoors breathing fresh air, visiting with the people he enjoyed talking to, and earning a few nickels each week. He loved this independence.

In only a short period of time, Elliott had formed some deep friendships with some of the staff at Sunland. His adopted "Papa Hatch" was head of maintenance, and he encouraged Elliott to help

115

him during the day or watch while he and his crew were undertaking heavy maintenance jobs. Elliott absorbed much of what these men knew about tools and equipment. His mind was eager to learn, even though he had always been indifferent to what was taught in the classroom.

My parents were greatly relieved by Elliott's happy adjustment. The dream they had before Elliott left for Farm Colony was coming true. He was happy, safe, and accepted. They had no need to feel guilty that he was no longer living with us.

Sunland at Miami was being built during the two years Elliott spent at Fort Myers. When my mother and I returned from a vacation in Mexico City, we learned that the new Sunland had opened and that Elliott was to be moved the following week.

His cottage, called "Harney," housed twenty boys. The furnishings were plain, but at least they were new. However, the cottage needed drapes, bedspreads, tablecloths, lamps, flowers, and some decorative touches to make it a home. The center boasted an administration building, a hospital, a developmental evaluation building, a schoolhouse, a chapel, a large cafeteria, and a maintenance building. The idea was to provide as much normalcy for the residents as possible. My parents were exultant! After so many years of desperately waiting and hoping for something, which had seemed in vain, their prayers were finally answered . . .or so they believed.

The concept was truly well conceived and the buildings were beautiful. Their Sunland parent group worked to make each cottage a home for their children. After all those years, my mother's interest in active involvement had never waned, and so nobody should have been surprised when she served as the first president of that parent group. As before, Elliott became one of the center's official messengers. His bicycle gave him many hours of relaxation and valuable exercise. His small stature, his thin smooth-shaven face, and his modern eyeglass

frames helped create the illusion of a 16-year-old boy, when in fact
Elliott was already a man in his late twenties. He could always be seen
at a distance from the road as one entered Sunland, peddling on his big
bike as if he were a normal suburban child.

His friendliness has always enabled him to meet practically
all of the parents who visited their children on weekends and to make
friends with a many of the 600 dedicated employees who staffed the
center. But Elliott's warmth was not restricted to adults. He made
friends with the boys in his cottage, as well as with some of the 1,000
clients in surrounding cottages.

But not everything was perfect. Elliott had his moments of heartbreak.
It was a story of young love. Mary was a beautiful young girl and
a victim of mild cerebral palsy. She was almost normal, except
for her slight speech and walking impairments. She was very kind
to Elliott. He adored her and lived from day to day for the time
he would see her. When they shopped on Sundays, Elliott always
wanted my mother to buy a gift for Mary. But after a short period of
rehabilitation, Mary was able to adjust to the outside world and get a
job, consequently leaving the center and Elliott forever. Mary leaving
was a shattering blow to Elliott. He had hoped to marry her some day.
After the initial shock, my mother explained to Elliott that marriage
entailed responsibilities and that he couldn't get married unless he
could support a wife. After Mary's departure, Elliott made numerous
acquaintances among the girls, and although he seems to have had
several crushes, to this day, no one has ever replaced Mary in his heart.

Despite his disappointment over Mary's departure, all in all,
things went smoothly for Elliott at Fort Myers. We visited him once a
month and usually took him to a motel overnight and part of Sunday.
He looked well and since he spent a great deal of time outdoors, he
had developed a radiant suntan.

During this time, my mother became involved in the fund-

117

raising group, Silver Disco, for the Dade County Association
for Retarded Citizens. She also became a charter member of the
Sunflower Society, whose charitable purpose was disabled and
handicapped people. Jean and my mother chaired their Psychic Dinner
and Dance. I did all the artistic work on the invitations and table
centerpieces, and private booths were provided for the seven psychics
who volunteered their services. The event was a huge success and we
managed to raise several thousand dollars.

A small group of our friends went on a weekend cruise. My father
loved this type of travel. His vacations now only included cruises.
After going on five cruises, my mother decided that she'd rather stay
on land, so my father found a boat mate in Uncle Julius. My father
usually closed the pharmacy for Christmas week when business was
slow and cruised at that time. It was relaxing for him because he
didn't have to catch any planes.

Elliott continued to make great progress working in the
carpenter shop. He made several footstools, which he gave to friends
as gifts. He derived a lot of pleasure from making things and giving
them away. He was still the official messenger for the center, taking
mail and messages from one department to another on his tricycle.
He also spent a lot of time with the center's doctor. He constantly
complained of headaches or stomachaches just so he could visit the
doctor. It gave him another person with whom to communicate.
Although this was not the existence my mother had envisioned for
Elliott when he was born, he had finally found himself living a stable
and satisfying life.

When summer ended, I entered the seventh grade at
Shenandoah Junior High School, which was only a half a block from
our home. Maxine's family had moved into a larger home in Coral
Cables, but it didn't take me long to form new friendships and become

118

involved in school activities. My mother filled her days with the trading stamp collection projects, which took up a good portion of her time. Trading stamps were not the same as greenback dollars, but for her they were preferable for buying a variety of equipment that Elliott and his fellow residents needed.

Sunland employed a highly qualified professional staff of all disciplines related to the mentally retarded and sufficient personnel to give them the proper care and training in an atmosphere of love and understanding. Many residents at Sunland were rehabilitated completely back into society.

The modern, central air-conditioned center had 53 buildings to implement a program, which was considered among the very best in existence. It was constructed on 240 acres of land and resembled a college campus.

While the State of Florida supplied the basic needs for Sunland, donations from groups and individuals paid for much of the equipment and special programs, which were enjoyed by the residents. To a great extent, it was these special additions that helped to accelerate the progress of these men and woman.

To my parents, the state had decided that Superintendent Dr. John Presley was going to be transferred to Miami to head the newest center in the state's system. Dr. Presely believed that the development and training of the child took first precedence over any other considerations. A special meeting was called for all interested parents to help select the names of the new cottages. The decision was to use the names of the past Presidents of the United States.

The first residents transferred from Fort Myers were from Dade, Broward, and Palm Beach counties. We were thrilled that Elliott was moving to South Florida and of course he was excited to being so close to home. It meant that we could visit him on Sundays and that he could come home for all the holidays and other time he

119

wanted. It was a warm feeling for our small family.

The first important thing on the agenda was the formation of the organization called Parents and Friends of Sunland. Never one to sit back and just watch, my mother became the association's first president and remained in office for the next eleven years.

The first important project requested by Dr. Presley was the needed equipment for the industrial workshop to provide sheltered employment for 200 trainees. The state was unable to provide this need, but they built the space for the facility. The state funded the buildings, beds, staff, and food, but the comfort items to create a more home-like atmosphere had to come from the public. My mom's organization raised the initial $1500 and presented it as the first installment with other monies being raised for the center.

Elliott again named himself as the official "greeter." He would park his bike near the entrance of the facility and direct the Sunday visitors to their prospective cottages. In that manner, Elliott became friends with many of the parents and visitors. He also became the official mail deliveryman, responsible for delivering mail from one office or department to another. It gave Elliott the opportunity to spend lots of time outdoors. In the new workshop, Elliott quickly resumed his passion for carpentry. He made small footstools, podiums, picture frames, and many other items.

Merchants Green Stamps provided free publicity for the first stamp drive which netted a dozen television sets valued at $150.00; each in exchange for 49 filled books of stamps. Once the stamps were collected, they were pasted into books. If they were loose, they were placed in deposit with the stamp company. Stamp accounts were much like bank accounts in those days. They saved and withdrew the books as they needed them in order to purchase gifts and assorted necessary equipment. Through a stamp broker they traded a variety of donated stamps for the one brand they were saving. The $2,000 electric organ cost 650 books and the 26 air conditioners were 100 books each.

All of these items added up to about $30,000, which they never could have raised in cash. Fortunately, my mother found that during the winter season, tourists in the area would give away stamps they were not saving back home. The Matron of the Order of the Amaranth, with its 3500 members, adopted the project as their own and they provided invaluable assistance in the stamp collecting drives.

Around this time, my mother was featured in the *Miami Herald* with a picture of her wearing a huge collar made of trading stamps. She was named the biggest stamp collector in Miami and the heading read "A New Charity Force." The paper asked for readers to help by sending their stamps or books to her address. She was swamped with the results and had to organize a committee to paste the stamps in books and trade off the books that they could not use.

Meanwhile, Elliott's problems had become less pronounced over the years. He only flared up and lost self-control on rare occasions when someone excited or teased him, but Elliott was living in comfortable and cheerful surroundings, and so such problems were rare.

All the boys in Elliott's cottage called my mother "mama." They always greeted her each Sunday with, "Hello, Mama" and shook her hand to say "goodbye" when she left. Elliott's last words were always, "Mom, can you leave me a dollar?" My mother loved leaving him not just one dollar, but two or three, knowing he was happy there and that it gave him joy to have some money in his pocket.

Our Elliott was fortunate. His cottage was occupied by high-level boys with whom he could interact. And even though the state required only a high-school education from the employees, many could easily play the "father" role and soon became "daddy" to the boys. Some residents whose parents visited infrequently were often taken home by these cottage parents to their own homes for weekend visits. To my mother's delight, Elliott's cottage had grown into somewhat of a close-knit family. And because Elliott had become so verbal and personal, was now making friends quite easily. One friend was Ralph, the maintenance supervisor. In fact, Ralph became like an uncle to Elliott, occasionally taking Elliott home to spend time with his family.

One day my mother decided to contact the nineteen other mothers from Harney cottage. They met on a Sunday afternoon to collect funds for new drapes for the windows, furniture for the day room, pictures for the walls, and floral arrangements to help make the new cottage in Miami look more like a home. Many other cottages decided to follow their example.

Every Sunday afternoon, my parents and our white poodle Collette, spent time with Elliott. A new shopping center had opened close to Sunland. Elliott enjoyed his treats from the ice cream fountain, and sometimes he would shop for sundry items he needed. Elliott was seeing the outside world and having new experiences. This was more knowledge than all the books at school could teach him. His learning disabilities had been recognized too late. Unfortunately for Elliott and his peers, there was a lack of knowledge regarding how to deal with victims of cerebral palsy, and sadly, this situation has yet to be fully rectified, for each year a thousand more like him are being born into the world and thrust upon a system that isn't quite sure what to do with them.

Rose Stosic, one of the mothers, was employed as the instructor of the arts and crafts room. Selected residents who could benefit from her talents were able to come to her class. She initiated the Greeting Card Recycling Project to bring in extra revenue to the center, after which, a concentrated drive for used greeting cards took place. With proper publicity in the area newspapers, thousands of cards were brought in or mailed to the center. The project then enabled the residents to cut the cards apart and paste the front and greeting on lightweight paper to become a new greeting card. A printed stamp was placed on the inside showing that they were made at Sunland, Miami. The cards were placed in packages of 12 and sold for $1.00. The demand was great, as they were much cheaper than the ordinary cards from the traditional card shops. This project lasted several years, until Rose retired and her daughter moved to a group home.

During the years of the crafts class, my mother was instrumental in securing pastries, cakes and cookies from the Andalusia Bakery in Coral Gables. Before the bakery closed each Saturday at 7 o'clock, my mother was permitted to pick up half of the leftover baked goods to take to Sunland on Sunday morning. They were delivered to the kitchen to be transferred to the art room on Monday morning. The residents were able to enjoy them for snacks for several days. If the supply was too large, the extra food was distributed in the cafeteria. This routine lasted until the craft department was eliminated for budget reasons.

Another important activity series at Sunland was the Jewish religious classes that were held each Sunday morning under a new Tikvah program sponsored by the Southeast Region of United Synagogues of America. All Jewish holidays were celebrated at the appropriate times by the holiday committee. Passover dinner was one of the favorite holidays. Most of the Jewish parents were very cooperative. They were like a family. The atmosphere at Sunland was very close-knit and informal. Many of the parents were very friendly with the superintendent and staff, and together they worked for the residents, striving to create a sense of community and togetherness that could never be accomplished without their efforts.

Then on May 10, 1971 a most memorable event at Sunland took place. It was a group Bar Mitzvah for ten young Jewish men, including Elliott. "Today you are a man." This familiar commendation, which concludes the Bar Mitzvah ceremony, is the cherished goal of most Jewish boys at age thirteen. When it comes well into adulthood, as it has for these fine young men today, there is a particularly keen sense of fulfillment, said Rabbi Solomon Schiff, director of the chaplaincy service of the Greater Miami Jewish Federation. Ten young men, the oldest being 45, demonstrated their knowledge of the Torah as a qualification for taking on the responsibility of adult Jewish life. Although it was the culmination of three years of study, their knowledge was very limited, and so was the responsibility those men were able to take in the Jewish community because of their mental and physical handicaps. But it was an emotional service, with families and school friends looking on in the Sunland Chapel.

So many of these boys have such a feeling of inadequacy, (as do many of their parents) but this event gave them a feeling that they are the same as others. It gave them a sense of fulfillment that they could never have achieved in sports or scholastic activities. The Bar Mitzvah certificate each boy received was exactly the same as the certificate any other 13-year-old boy received upon completing the course of study and publicly demonstrating his grasp of the foundations of Jewish life. The boys were also presented with a beautiful silver-encased prayer book, which Elliott has cherished ever since. This was an example of the federation's philosophy that the Jewish community believes that the individual—no matter who he or she is—is the rarest, most precious capital resource of our society.

Many Hebrew songs were sung and several prayers chanted. Song sheets were distributed so that everyone could partake in the ceremony. A lavish reception provided by the Parent group in the employee cafeteria followed the services. Publicity in the *Miami Herald* brought the event to the attention of synagogues and the public throughout the South Florida community.

In the fall of 1971, my father decided to retire. His health was failing, and even though he wanted to continue working, he had no choice. His surgery from minieres had taken its toll, leaving him with the removal of one ear and left him relying upon a hearing aid in the other. My father's retirement was very emotional for both of my parents. My mother curtailed all of her volunteer work to keep him company. Collette, our wonderful little poodle, was constantly at his side. My father spent time visiting his sisters, Sadie and Esther.

During this time, I was completing my last two years at the University of Florida in Gainesville where I was studying interior design and architecture. In stark contrast to Elliott, whom I'm sure would have been equally successful were it not for his terrible condition, I always excelled academically. Of course my mother loved both her children dearly, but in light of all her struggles and disappointments with Elliott, I had been a particularly rich source of joy and hope, and my very existence has helped sustain my mother in the good times and bad.

I can undoubtedly say that I reattributed my mother's unconditional love with respect, admiration, and followed her unique actions of always helping the less fortunate.

Chapter 8
How Elliott Changed My Life

I was always scared about telling my friends that I had a handicapped brother. I was concerned if anyone I would date in my future relationships will be affected by my brother's condition. Up graduation in 1973 from the University of Florida I got a job with the prestigious Architectural Firm of Ferendino Grafton Spillis & Candela in Coral Gables. Even though I wanted to avoid anything medical in my career, one of my first projects was to design The Children's Clinic at Bascom Palmer Eye Institute in The Medical Center Campus at The University of Miami. I did such a good job understanding with the design that I was rewarded with another medical job.

My second project was Miami Dade Community College Medical Center Campus. Because of my involvement the project's interiors, my firm won an award from the IBD (Institute of Business Designers).

My mother raised the money to renovate the cafeteria where my brother lived at the Sunland Training Center in Miami and I brought the job to the firm where I worked, Ferendino Grafton Spills & Candela in Coral Gables.

By now all the people that I worked with knew that I had a handicapped brother and they not only accepted the fact but encouraged me with their support for my work.

In 1975 I got married to a lawyer, Rick Mattaway his brother in law, Stuart was an OBGYN doctor and had an understanding of Cerebral Palsy. Pam and Stuart as well as their 5 kids always included Elliott in all the family functions.

In 1979 we purchased a 2 story Chinese Village home in Coral Gables. Although we where concerned that Elliott would not be able to climb to the second floor he was able to come every Thanksgiving and Christmas for 11 years and celebrate with us and stay at the upstairs bedroom. After 15 years Rick and I got divorced and at 40 years old I found myself dating wondering who would accept my handicapped brother.

As my divorce was being finalized, I met again an architect that I worked with at Ferendino Grafton since 1973. He helped me with the final stages of my divorce and ended up getting married sooner thereafter. Albert J. Socol is the best thing that ever happened to me since not only accept my brother became my partner and best friend.

Albert included Elliott while we were dating and took him to the movies and made arrangements for him to go to Disneyworld with our housekeeper and husband.

We also took him to Universal Studious in Orlando, Florida, but Elliott was scared of most rides. Because for Elliot the most important thing is family, we bring him home for his birthday in September and in January to visit with his cousins from Pittsburg and his Uncle Ed in Sarasota, Florida. Uncle Ed gave him a T shirt with the name of Ed's store Kane's Furniture that is Elliott's favorite shirt to wear.

After each visit Elliott always calls me and thanks us for taking him out and what is good time he had.

Elliott makes me appreciate life and thankful for what life gave me. I also value my relationship with my husband and my friends and better understand what my mother went through with Elliott's handicapped.

We almost lost Elliot when he had gallbladder surgery in 2003 the same operation that killed my father in 1973. Elliott was invited to my stepson wedding in Naples, Florida but could not attend because of his operation. From the wedding we rushed to the hospital in Hollywood, Florida thankfully he survived and today at 70 years old he is still active visiting his friends. Recently he became friends with a neighbor named Caitlin who is 17 years old and Elliott calls his girlfriend. Elliott always calls me to ask for a gift for Caitlin. He is always considerate and thoughtful and bears no negative thoughts about his condition or bad feeling for anybody. He has lived in Woodhouse for 32 years where he has his own work shed that my mother bought and equipped for him with different tools that Elliott uses to repair and build things.

Since my mother passed away in 2003 Goodwill has a program that gets him and the other 15 handicapped adults, out everyday to bowling, picnics, movies, etc.

On Saturday he shares a taxi with 3 other handicapped adults and goes to downtown Hollywood and "has a ball".

On Sunday he goes to church with one of the neighbors and even though he was born Jewish I told him that "God will listen to his prayers".

Chapter 9
Monthly Visits to Dania

I promised my mother that I would get my brother and visit with him at least once a month. I fulfill my promise and take Elliott out to eat, visit a Museum or look at the old neighborhood. Everyday I get several calls from Elliott. He says "Hello sweetheart, when are you coming to see me", even if we just had took him out the day before.

We also look forward to the visit with Elliott and go to several places; some new and some old and it constitutes a mini vacation. Albert quizzes Elliott about the manufacturer of the rental car we are driving and for sure he knows the brand and vehicle type. He loves to go out to eat and I feed him with the same love that my mother did for so many years.

In May 2002, I started Recycled Arts with my dear friend, Marie Spafford, where we got the fabrics donated from the Design Center in Dania, Florida, and she took it to her school where she teaches, Corkscrew Middle School, and the sewing teacher Loretta had the students make pillows, quilts, tote bags, etc.

All the items were then sold and the funds went to "Project Elliott" at Woodhouse.

Gloria Dixon, the head of the Woodhouse Dania operations has been there for over 30 years and done a magnificent job taking care of Elliott.

I remember that when my mother passed away she insisted that Elliott be present at the cemetery, she showed up with Elliott, whom she dressed up in a beautiful dark suit.

My husband kids with me that my mother made me into a monster that knows everything because she knew that one day I would take over the responsibility for Elliott although he is a ward of the State. I perform those duties gladly and hope to do so for as long as Elliott is with us.

Chapter 10
Elliott's Own Story

When I was just a baby just before I learned to walk wile lying in my cradle I would try my best to talk it wasn,t long befor I talk and all the neughbors heard my folks were very proud of me for <u>Mother</u> was the word.

M is for the million things she game me
O is only that shes groing old.
T is for the tears she shed to save me.
H is for her heart of purest gold.
E is for her eyes with love light shining.
R is right and right she'll always be.
Put them all together they spell <u>MOTHER</u>
A word that means the world to me.

Elliott S. Weiss

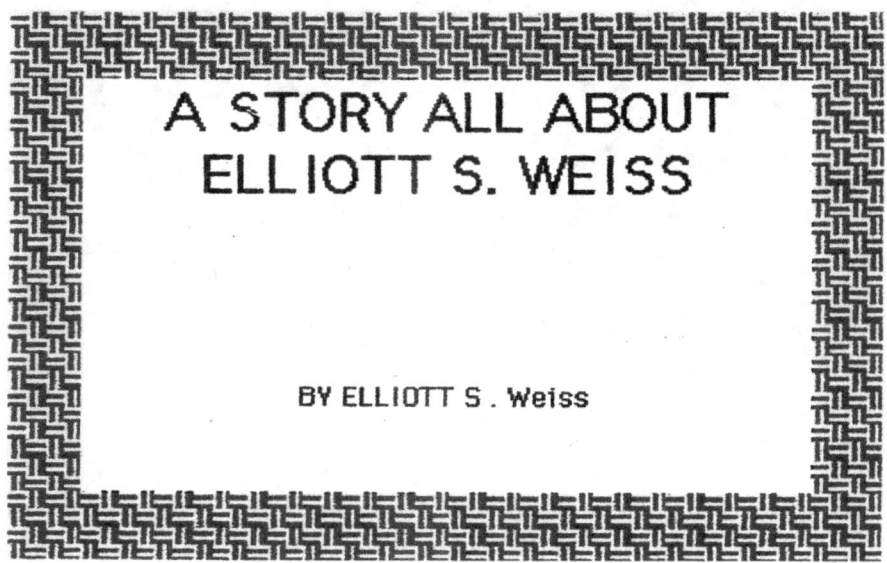

A STORY ALL ABOUT ELLIOTT S. WEISS

BY ELLIOTT S . Weiss

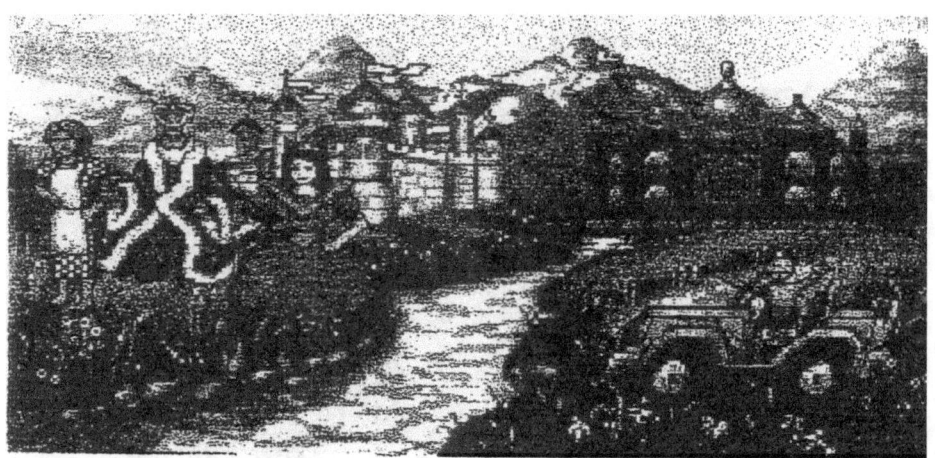

I was born in California Pa. One day my uncle came over to my house and took me for a ride in a Jeep from the army. He was an M.P. I was dressed in my Navy suit then.

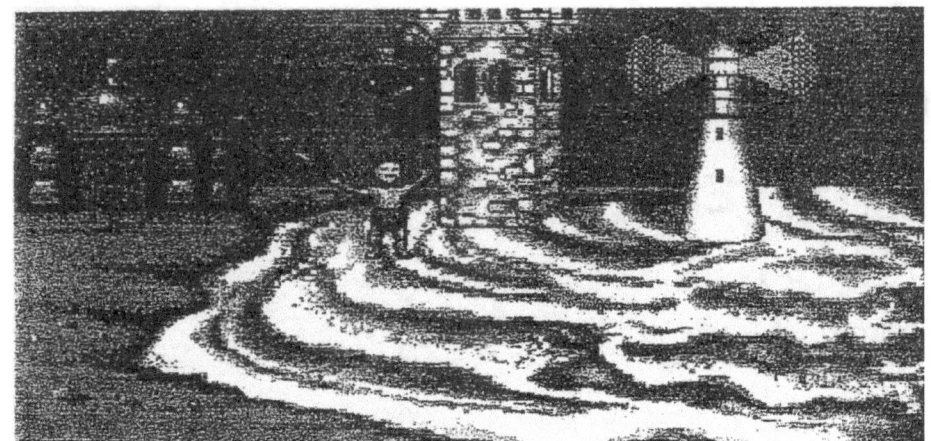

I came to Miami in 1940 from California Pennsylvania for my
health. I did not walk or talk. Mother and Mary and I came down.
We had a bad storm. We had no lights so we were in the dark.
Mother, Mary and Grandpa lived with us then.

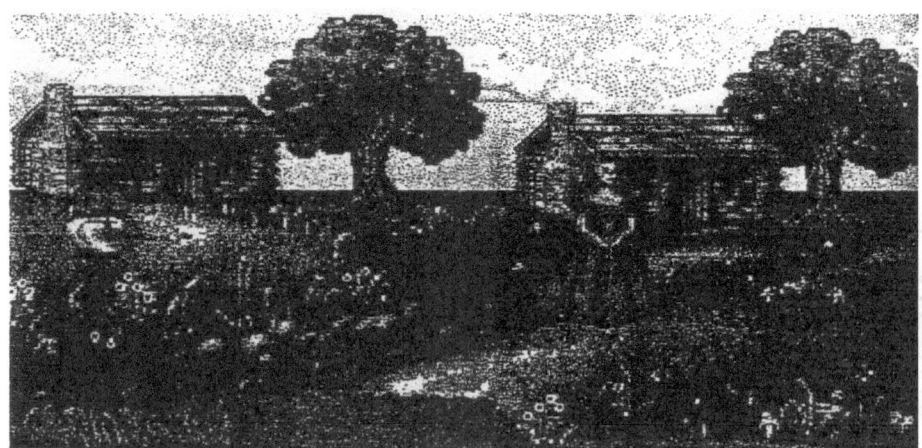

I came from Pennsylvania to Miami for my health. I did not
walk or talk, so Uncle Bill made me a walker out of 2x4's.
It had big wheels on it. We had a bad storm then. We were out of
power.

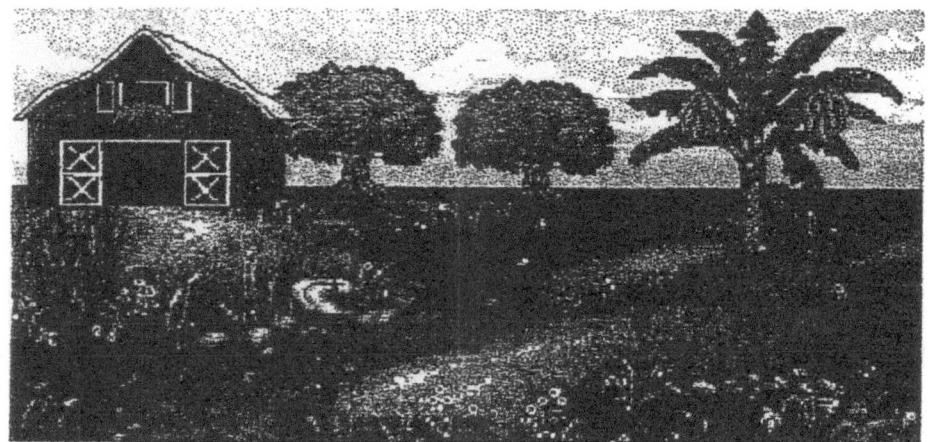

I moved to Pompano. There I met and fell in love with my baby
nurse. She took care of me. Her name was Marty Holiday. She took
care of me when I was small. We would have sweet buns and boy
were they good. On Wednesdays we had dounuts.

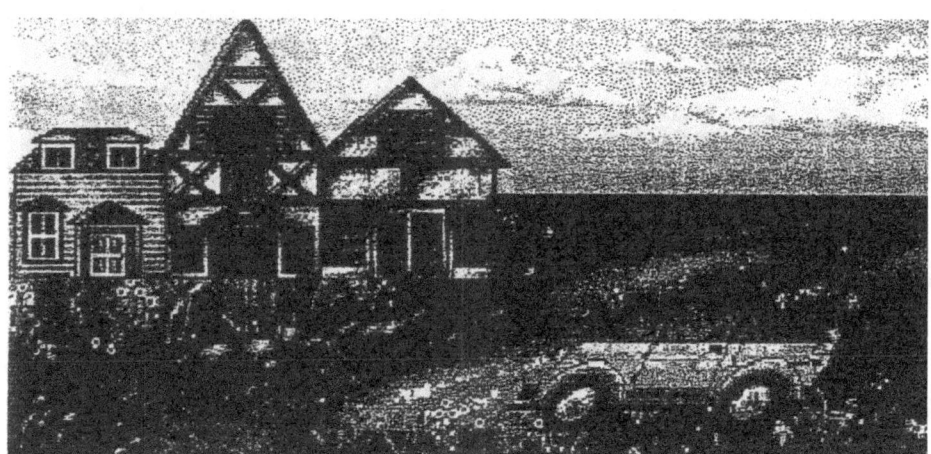

After two years, my mother and aunt and uncle came and
took me home. I was in Pompano at the time. Uncle Ben had a
green convertable. They came to take me home.

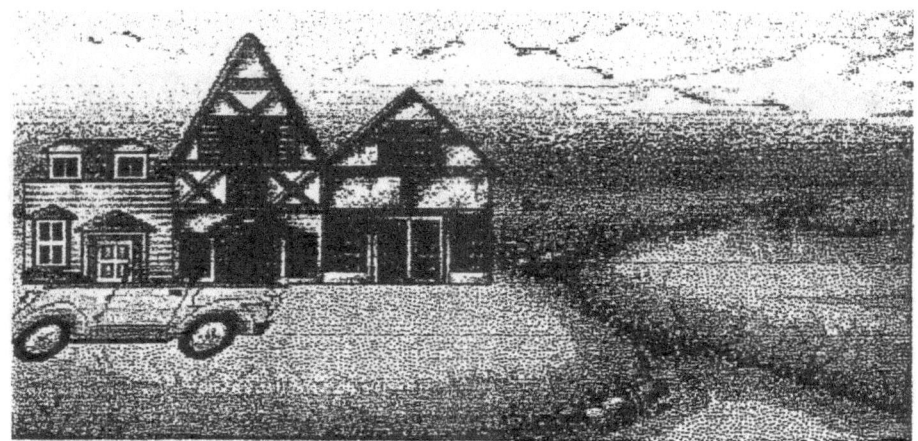

I moved to Miami. I went to a day school called Miramar. I rode a
limosene to school every day. The firemen came every week and
took us up four flights of stairs to the movies. Then I moved
from Miramar to Roosevelt School.

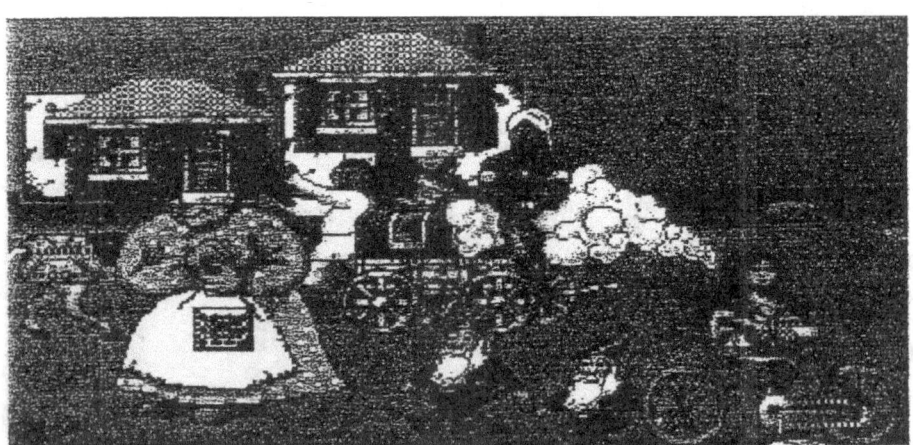

I went to the Ringling Brothers Barnun and Baily Circus
every year. We would take a day off from school. The Shriners
and Police would make a day of it. Abe Goldman was a Shriner.
I had a bus driver. Her name was Vera Cole.

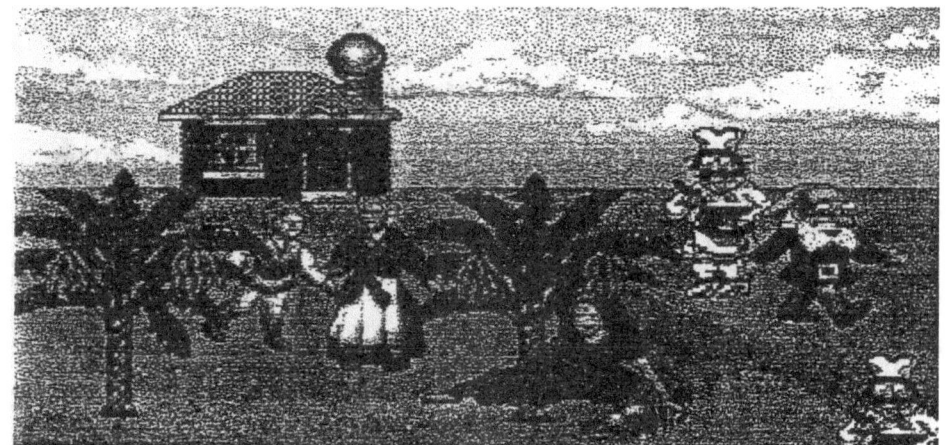

Then I moved to a high school called Ada Merrit. There I met
a pal of mine. His name was Bobby Brawn. His mom drove me
to U.C.P. from Ada Merrit. I met my old OT teacher from my
old school. Her name was Mrs. McArther.

My teacher was Mrs. Mcarther, wife of Mr. Mcarther. One day
we went to the dairy and saw how they put the milk in the
cartons and they showed us through the plant. We had lunch and
came back to school.

Then I moved to Ada Merritt. One day when I came home from
school, my Aunt and my baby nurse me at the bus stop and said,
"Let's go get Mother from the hospital." Then I went in the house
and saw Mother and Marlene. Boy was I happy.

My father was a pharmasist down town at 1431 N. Bay Shore
Drive. Then I went to UCP of Miami. I took 2 busses every day.
Some days I would get a ride home by a lady who had a son that
went to the center every day. His mom would take me home. His
name was Presten Lustig.

I had an uncle Dave who was a judge in Pittsburgh. My mom
started U.C.P.because of me.

One day when I came home from school my Aunt Tilly and Mary met me at the bus stop and said, "Let's go and get Mother from the Hospital." So I went in the house and saw Mother and Marlene. They were pulling my leg.

My father had a Pharmacy in Miami. It was in downtown Miami at 1431 North Bay Shore Drive. I had an uncle who was a judge in Pittsburgh. His name was Dave H. Weiss.

Then I moved to Sunland in Gainsville. It was like being in the army. Every one wore Army green.

Then I moved to Ft. Myers. There I met a nice man. His name was Ira C. Hatch. Boy what a good time I had with him. We made a train from nothing. We used old air line luggage carts and built a train. It took four days to build a coach. The engine was an airport tracter. We had a big store on the train. It was called the Mini Mart on wheels. Then I was a messenger boy in Fort Myers and a shoe man.

My mother started U.C.P. because of me. One day the Schriners had a Easter egg party and they unvailed a big bus at the Easter egg hunt.

I am a member of the Harlum Globetrotters team.

I saw the Glenn Miller band at Leghi Acers.

I did not walk so my uncle made me a big walker out of 2x4s and big wheels. They did not think of all things like they have today.

One year I gave Miss Sophie Tucker an Easter Lilly.

One day Mrs. Huggins said to me, "How would you like to suprise your mother?" So I said, "O.K." So we went down to W.I.O.D. and had a party for my mother on mothers day and sang the Mother's day song.

I had a teaacher by the name of Mrs. Jones. She had no hands. I want to thank Mr. Fred P Hicky for helping me with my book.

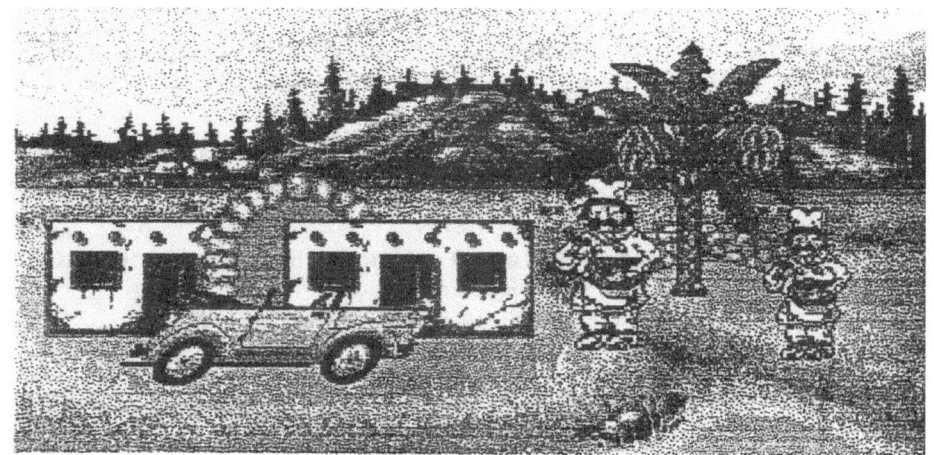

Then I moved to Birmingham to Charlanne school. The school
was on a big hill, at 1019 Oxmore Rd. Birmingham, Ala.
I met a girl friend. She lived off grounds in Alabama.
Big Rose and Ema Jean were the cooks in Alabama.

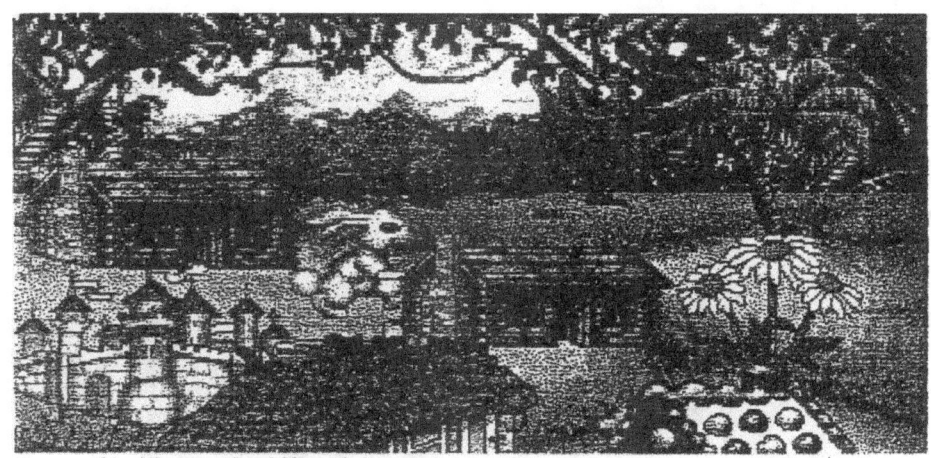

From Ft. Myers to Miami I road in a big stake truck with Papa
Hatch. We made one stop at the Old South Bar B Q. From there
we came to Sunland. There I met more friends, and I walked
through Hurricane Dona when she blew through Miami.

I met Robert Q. Louis at the first Telethon for U.C.P., and boy, the food they had in the back! Then I moved from Sunland to Woodhouse in Dania. There I met a dear friend called Gloria Dixin and I have loved her ever since.

I have my own work shop on the patio. I could live out there. It is so peacefull there. We have a God Father. His name is Frank Hill and my mom is our God Mother.

I just met a fireman. His name is Robert Hazen and boy what a good friend. What a good friend.

We have a great staff. We go to camp Challenge in the summer time. It is like my second home because the staff treats me very well. At Woodhouse we have a lot of fun at parties. We went to Disnsy World 3 times.

I will not forget going to Aunt Sadie's on Sunday and having stuffed cabbage and Aunt Ester's for spaghetti.

Yours truely, Elliott S. Weiss

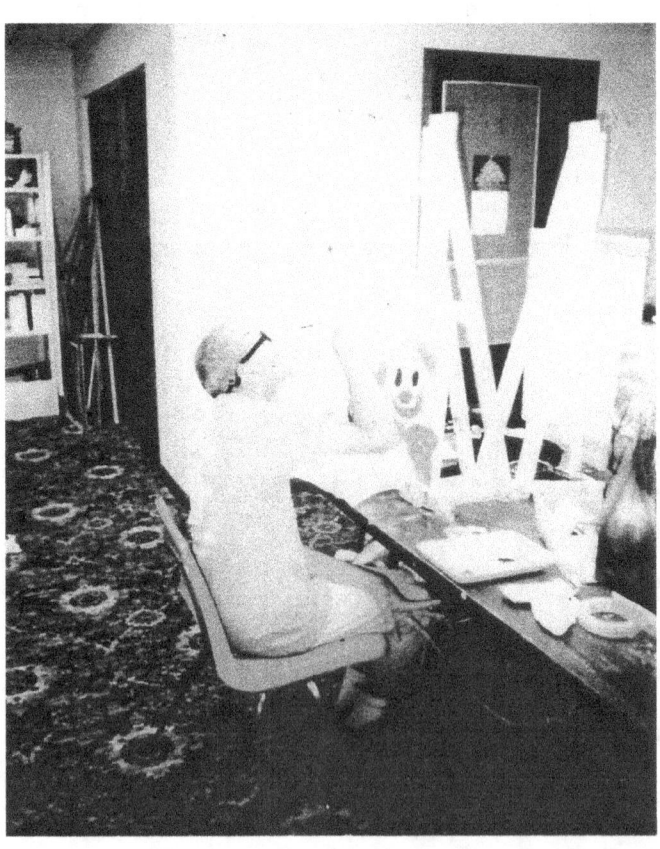

Chapter 11
What is available today for CP

I did not have any children in my first or second marriages because of a medical condition that was not uncovered until last January 2004. The irony is that now I could have children, but it is too late for my biological clock.

But, I often wonder, what if history would have repeated what is available today for parents with children born with Cerebral Palsy.

Here's what I found out.
1. Dr Bernard Brucker Associate Professor and Director of the Bio Feedback. Laboratory at the University of Miami, Florida has developed a program he has applied to children as well as adults with brain damage. Over 30 years of research, Bio Feedback helped patients from all over the world and Dr. Brucker has seen and treated over 9,000 cases.

One of the most cases was featured in a movie with Jane Seymour "The Heart of Healing"

It is the story of a young girl from South Africa non-ambulatory, with no free standing balance. The doctors and therapists concluded that she would never be able to stand or walk. Dr. Brucker treated her once a year for three weeks over several years. Now she is independent and without the use of any devises recently ran a marathon.

Dr. Brucker sustains that although it is true that the brain cells are permanent and cell death, even at birth, is irrecoverable, his work has focuses on using specific learning methods to teach the use of alternative cells to take over the task of the destroyed cells in order to gain motor function.

2. Conductive Education.

Conductive Education was started in Budapest, Hungary, not far from where my father was born. It is a very intensive type of physical therapy and is getting very good results. I visited several times their facility in Ft. Lauderdale, FL and spoke with several parents who expressed their satisfaction with the progress that their children were making.

Conductive Education is now available throughout the whole United States.

3. Cord Blood Therapy

Dr. Joanne Kurtzberg at Duke University through Cord Blood Therapy has developed a cure for Cerebral Palsy. This happened in March 2008, she reintroduces the Cord Blood when the child is 2 years old and by the time they are 7 years old they are cured of Cerebral Palsy.

It is imperative to save your Cord Blood, it could save your child's life one day.

Dr. Diane Wilen
4806 Arthur St.
Hollywood, FL 33021

January 18, 2005

Dear Marlene:

As you know, I have been a psychologist with the Broward County School system for over 30 years. I was honored with an outstanding practice of school psychology award by the Florida Association of School Psychologists and the Phil Seat award from the Broward Association of School Psychologists.

I have known Elliott since I married my husband over 30 years ago. Elliott is my husband's cousin and he has watched our sons grow up.

Elliott has been an inspiration for my son Craig who is planning to go to medical school. We take Elliott out about once a month and include him in our annual Thanksgiving dinner.

Elliott always has a positive outlook and is very appreciative for whatever we do for him, and he especially loves being with his family. The simple things make him happy and he does not complain about his disabilities and what he cannot do. He calls all the time and though sometimes it is hard to understand him, somehow he manages to get the message across.

Elliott has been a very positive role model for our family. His kind words often make our day!

Love your cousin,

Diane

Diane

Suzanne Migdall
1515 SE 11 Street
Fort Lauderdale, FL 33316
Tel (954) 448-0549   Fax (954) 525-8122

January 22, 2005

Dear Marlene:

I have known Marlene for over forty years, since I was three years old and moved across the street from the Weiss family in Miami. As we grew up together, Aunt Rose, Marlene's Mother was like my second Mother, and we have remained close friends throughout our lives.

My family knew all the challenges that Rose Weiss had to face to educate Elliott and the public about cerebral palsy. Like Elliott, my Aunt Ada was born with cerebral palsy on September 5, 1916, in Philadelphia. When Ada Gordon was a year old they did not know what cerebral palsy was. She was told that she would not live past thirteen years old.

Aunt Ada is now 88 years old and is living a full life in South Beach. She married during her lifetime, learned another language, Spanish, and helped the Cuban refugees when they arrived in Miami. While Ada is confined now to a wheelchair, her outlook on life has been positive while she has helped many people.

Last year I had the privilege of meeting famed actress Mia Farrow whose book "A Memoir What Falls Away" covers her adoptions of many handicapped children, including a boy with cerebral palsy. In Farrow's New York Times bestseller book and during her lectures promoting her book, she is very enlightening about the many opportunities that are now available for children who are handicapped.

The public needs to be aware that handicapped people can lead productive lives. Rose Weiss spent her life devoted to the cause of raising awareness and funding for the handicapped. During my childhood she pioneered Sunland Training Center and the organization that funded it, the Sunflower Society. Rose was a real fighter for the handicapped and was tireless in her efforts to contribute to this cause.

As a Mother to Elliott, Rose was courageous in her battles to help the handicapped and her son. Elliott has been an inspiration to all that know him, his memory and intelligence continue to surpass his disabilities.

With love, your best friend and Sister,
Suzanne

Tobe Marmorstein
10903 S.W. 124th Road
Miami, Florida 33176
January 18, 2004

Dear Marlene,
I am writing to you, in response to your question about Elliott's education. I have known Elliott for over 40 years, I first met him when we were in High School. To me he looked pretty normal, but his speech was difficult to understand. Today, I am a Dade County Public school teacher with over 25 years in the field of Exceptional Education. I have taught students with Learning Disabilities, Educable Mentally Handicapped, Trainable Mentally Handicapped, and students who are Other Health Impaired.

Elliott would have been eligible for any one of these programs if he was attending public school today. IDEA (Individuals with Disabilities Educational Act) provides that all children with a disability, ages birth to 22, are entitled to a free and appropriate education. No public school is allowed to turn such children away from their doors. Today this federal law goes even further in it's attempt to "include" these students in the regular school program whenever it is deemed appropriate for the students overall goals.

Children and Adults with Cerebral Palsy vary in their abilities. Some people are only affected physically, others mentally and physically. I have a close friend, Debbie Marks, who works in the school system as a Transition Counselor; she has CP. She is a college graduate and helps exceptional education students transition from school to the community and work.

There are many opportunities for children with special needs today thanks to IDEA. Many of the local Publix markets employ students with disabilities, especially the mentally challenged. Many students go on to live in supported living situations or group homes. They are employed in our community or in sheltered workshops or attend activity centers so they do not sit at home idle all day, but become productive members of their community.

I hope I have answered your questions. Your Mom always did what was best for Elliott. She was always on the cutting edge of progress. I believe Elliott was one of the first to leave Sunland for a group home which back then was the emerging philosophy to provide more home-like conditions rather than the large institutions with their inherent problems. Her dedication and commitment and my exposure to your family, helped me to make teaching children with special needs my life long career.

Much Love,

Tobe

143

Publications
1941 - 2008

Time Magazine – February 17, 1941

Elliott's Doctor

From the hazards of embryonic life on the rough passage of birth, one out of some 1,000 children emerges with certain motor centres of his brain seriously damaged. If he matures, his central nervous system remains in an infantile state, like a telephone switchboard with crossed wires. Bombarded by sense impulses, he always gets the wrong number - brings the wrong muscles into play. Such children are victims of spastic paralysis. In walking, their toes scrape the ground, their legs cross if a scissors bend, and the touch of a finger may send them sprawling.

Although some of them drool like idiots, spastic children are usually of normal intelligence. Neither medicine nor surgery can cure them. Chief hope for them is to train the healthy fibres of the brain to take over the functions of injured sections. Shining example of such a self-helped spastic is Dr. Earl Reinhold Carlson* of Manhattan's Neurological Institute. Son of Swedish immigrants, iron-willed Dr. Carlson worked his way through the University of Minnesota and Princeton. A group of friends sent him to Yale Medical School. He has started a dozen schools for spastics all over the U.S., has helped 8,000 fellow sufferers to control their unruly muscles. This week, in a pithy little book (Born That Way; John Day; $1.75), he tells the story of his struggles.

Earl Carlson was born in Minneapolis during the blizzard of 1897. He was injured by forceps, and still bears a scar on his forehead. He had to crawl on all fours till he was five, but was robust and mischievous. One day, to his mother's amazement, little Earl's flailing arms stole some apples from a fruit stand. "It was the first time that my hand had ever done my bidding," he said. "My stolen apples gave me the clue, not followed up for years, that the secret of control for the muscularly handicapped lies in concentration on purpose."

Because his parents were poor, Earl was not coddled. When he was six, his mother "drove" him to school, where he suffered agonies. Grasping a pencil was for him what tightrope walking is to a normal man. Although he dared not eat in public till he was 18 or 19, he once picked the lock of his cousin's Model-T Ford with a hairpin, drove carefully around the block.

In 1918, while he was at college, Earl's mother died and the following year his father killed himself. Instead of going to pieces, the crippled orphan boy matured overnight. Today Dr. Carlson, happily married, spends summers in Manhattan and Long Island, winters in his school at Pompano, Fla. He speaks slowly, writes in a sprawling hand, but

cont.

dances, swims, paddles a canoe, is a good shot. Dr. Carlson deplores pampering for spastics, insists that only the rigors of life can teach them to teach themselves control.

Chief Maxim:
Physical training just for "motion sake" is useless. To develop, muscles must be used for a purpose. Spastic children must be sent to school as soon as possible. They must not have their lessons done for them, for they learn only by experience. Writing or typing, is very important, for muscular movements somehow help to fix facts in the spastic's brain.

"Born That Way" is the title of a book which the John Day Company has announced for publication on Feb. 13. The author is Dr. Earl R. Carlson, one of the leading practitioners in the treatment of the birth-injured. Dr. Carlson himself was so severely injured at birth that he has never had the full use of his muscles. Despite this handicap he obtained his medical degree, and during approximately a decade of practice has been consulted by more than eight thousand birth-injured persons or their parents. He has now told his story in a book which may serve as a guide and psychological spur to all handicapped persons.

* No kin to Chicago's Physiologist Anton Julius Carson (Time, Feb. 10).

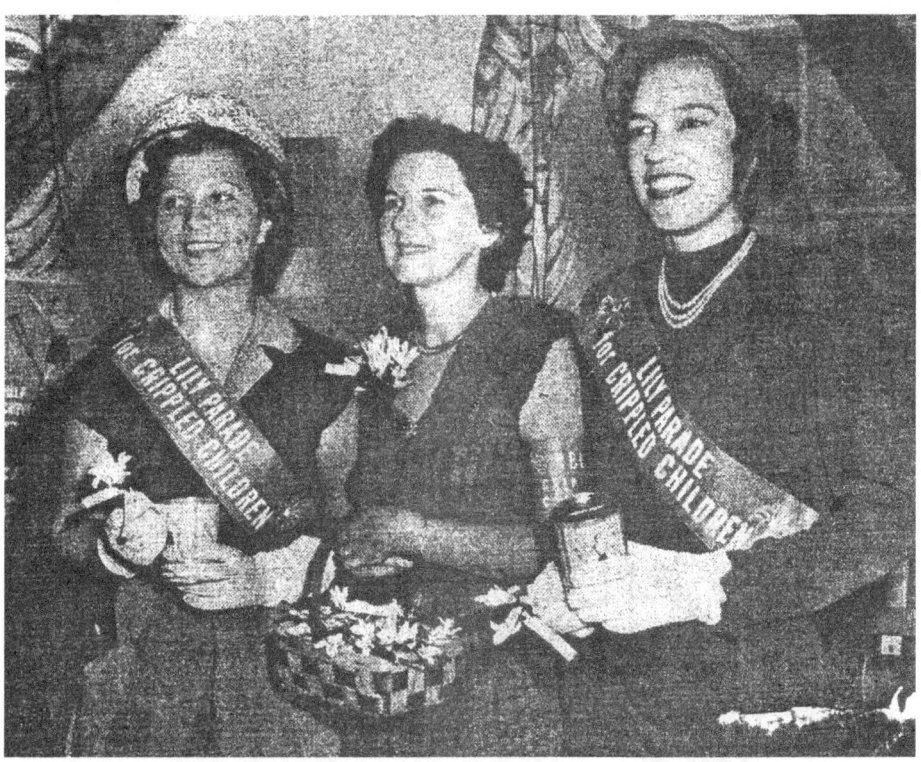

Aid to crippled children – Arrangements for the annual Easter lily tag day, April 3 of the Dade County Society for Crippled Children will be carried out by 40 member organizations and 300 volunteer workers. Left to right, Mrs. Edward F. Boardman, Miami Jaycee auxiliary; Mrs. Edward Weiss, tag day chairman; Mrs. Raymond L. Parker, Miami Junior Woman's club; were pictured at recent meeting, with tag day equipment.

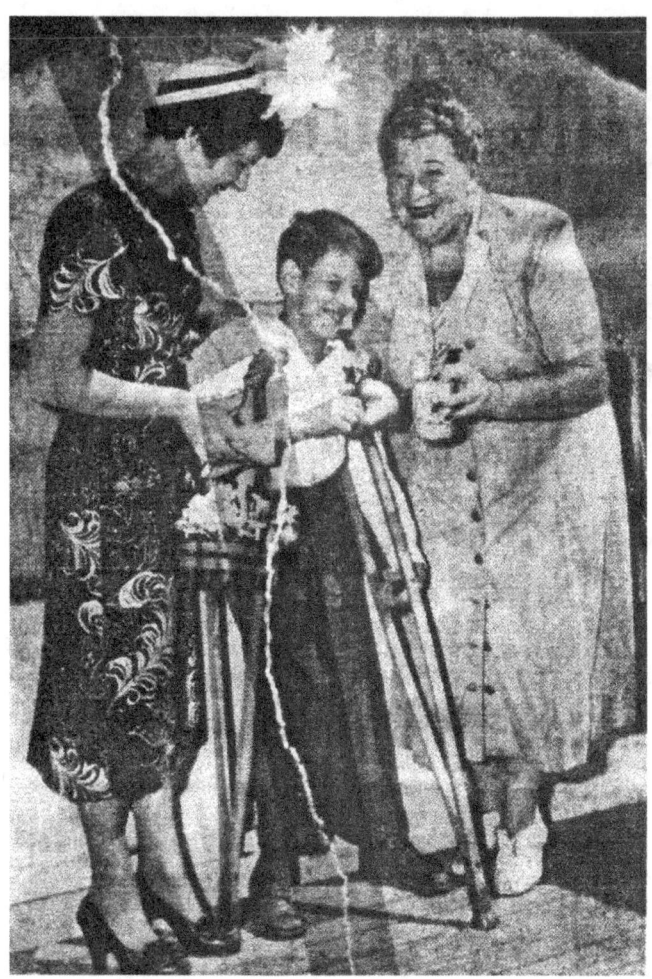

KNOWN AND LOVED for her interest in handicapped children, Sophie Tucker (right) is the first to buy a lily for the Dade County Crippled Children's Society's annual tag day, scheduled for Monday. Elliott Weiss, pupil at Roosevelt School for Exceptional Children (center) and his mother, Mrs. Edward Weiss, chairman of the drive, seem as happy with the transaction as Miami's noted visitor. Because of the interest in the campaign, a silver tea will be given Wednesday from 3 to 5 p.m. at the school, 5100 NE Second Ave. Guests will have the opportunity of touring the school.

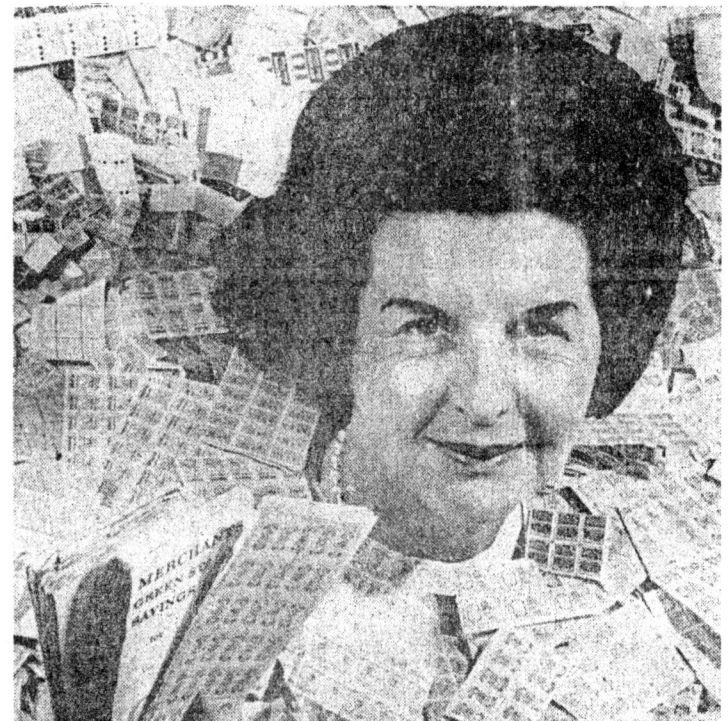

Greater Miami's Biggest Stamp Collector?
...Mrs. Edward Weiss sparks aid for Sunland Center

New Charity Force Stampbooks

AND what makes a stamp collector?

Mrs. Edward Weiss, 1900 SW 18th Ave., probably the biggest stamp collector in town, is the mother of a 24-year-old, cerebral palsied retardee at the Sunland Training Center in Fort Myers.

She and other Sunland parents are the kind of people who travel hundreds of miles on a hot, summer day to visit a child who is at once heartbreak and their greatest spur to action.

To Mrs. Weiss, action means trading stamps – millions of them.

Already she has masterminded the collection of about 1,000 books of trading stamps for television sets and an electric organ.

Now she's off and running to get 19 Sunland cottages air conditioned – two air conditioners to each cottage at 107 stamp books apiece.

At 1,500 stamps per book, that's 5,778,000 stamps.

The group has already donated 514 books worth of air conditioners for the Sunland nurseries, and another group in Palm Beach provided another five air conditioners.

"There's a lot of work connected with it," she said. "But as I gather more experience along the line, I am able to do more and get more from people."

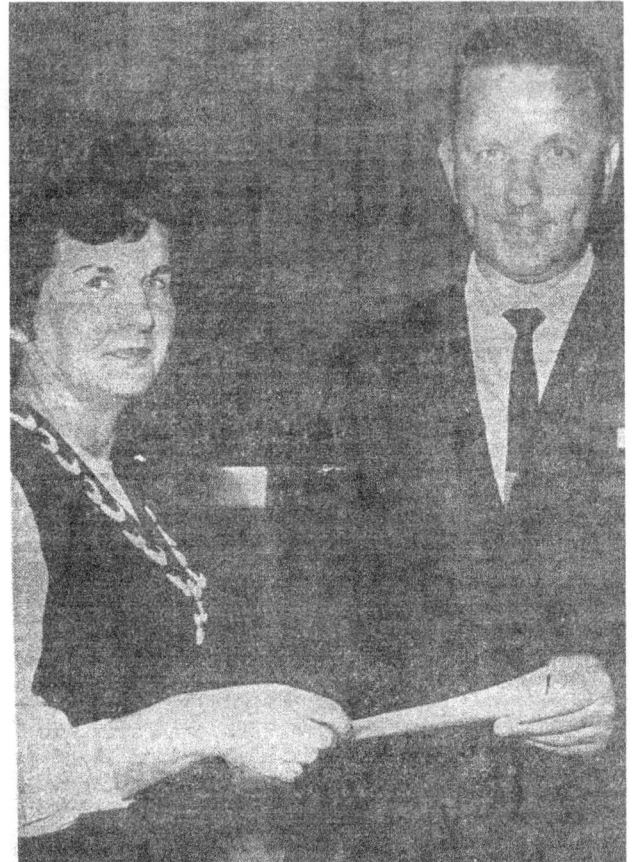

President Mrs. Edward Weiss Checks In With Dr. J. M. Presley

Sunland Training Center
Gets Check for $1,500

Parents and Friends of Sunland Training Center, Inc., presented a check for $1,500 to Dr. J. M. Presley, Superintendent of the new Miami's Sunland Training Center.

Dedicated to the welfare, health and happiness of retarded children the Center is located at 20000 NW 47th Ave.

The $1,500 is the first installment toward the purchase of equipment for an industrial workshop that will eventually provide sheltered employment for 200 trainees.

"The state provides funds for buildings, beds, staff and food, but the recreation and training items must come from the general public," says Mrs. Edward Weiss, president of the Parents and Friends group.

"Thousands more are needed to complete the workshop. Checks may be sent to Box 92, Opa Locka, Fla.," says Mrs. Weiss.

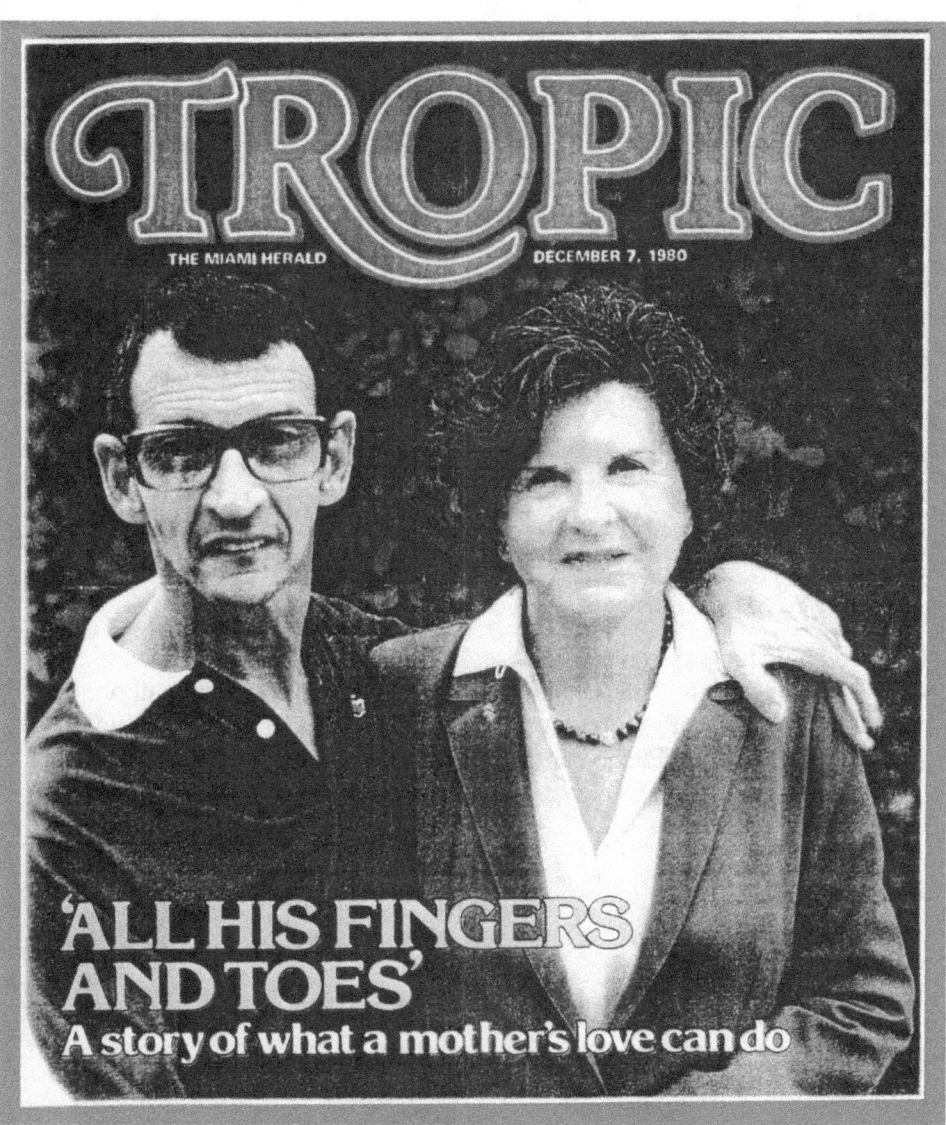

TROPIC

THE MIAMI HERALD DECEMBER 7, 1980

'ALL HIS FINGERS AND TOES'
A story of what a mother's love can do

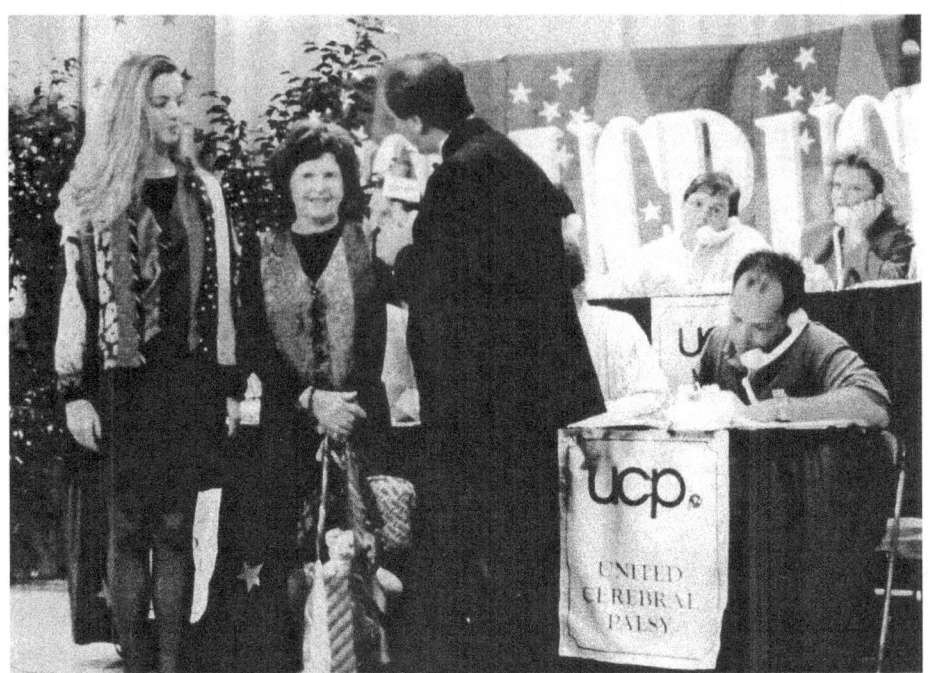

Family Ties

I still continue to work for Woodhouse. In August 1993, I organized a recycling project to use silk ties in making vests, hand-sewn, with all profits donated to the Recreation Fund for adult clients at Woodhouse" Cerebral Palsy Adult Home in Dania. Each year they are able to enjoy a weekend at a motel near Orlando. After two weeks of camp session, adequate monies were raised in 1993-94.

Elliott is now 55 years old. He still lives at Woodhouse. He has his own workshop in back of the patio. At work, he has learned to operate a computer. He rides a three-wheel bike and motorized scooter.

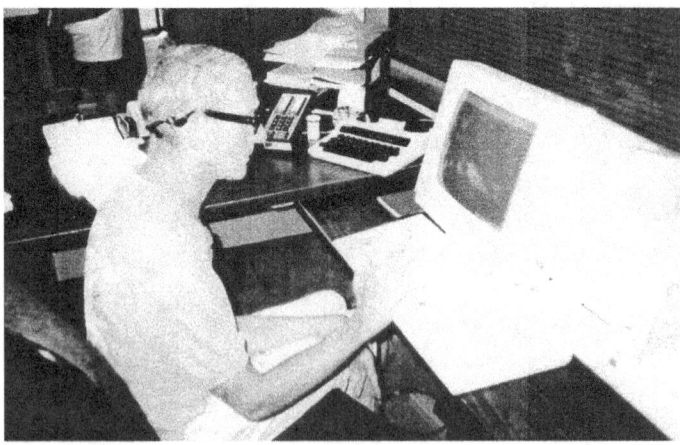

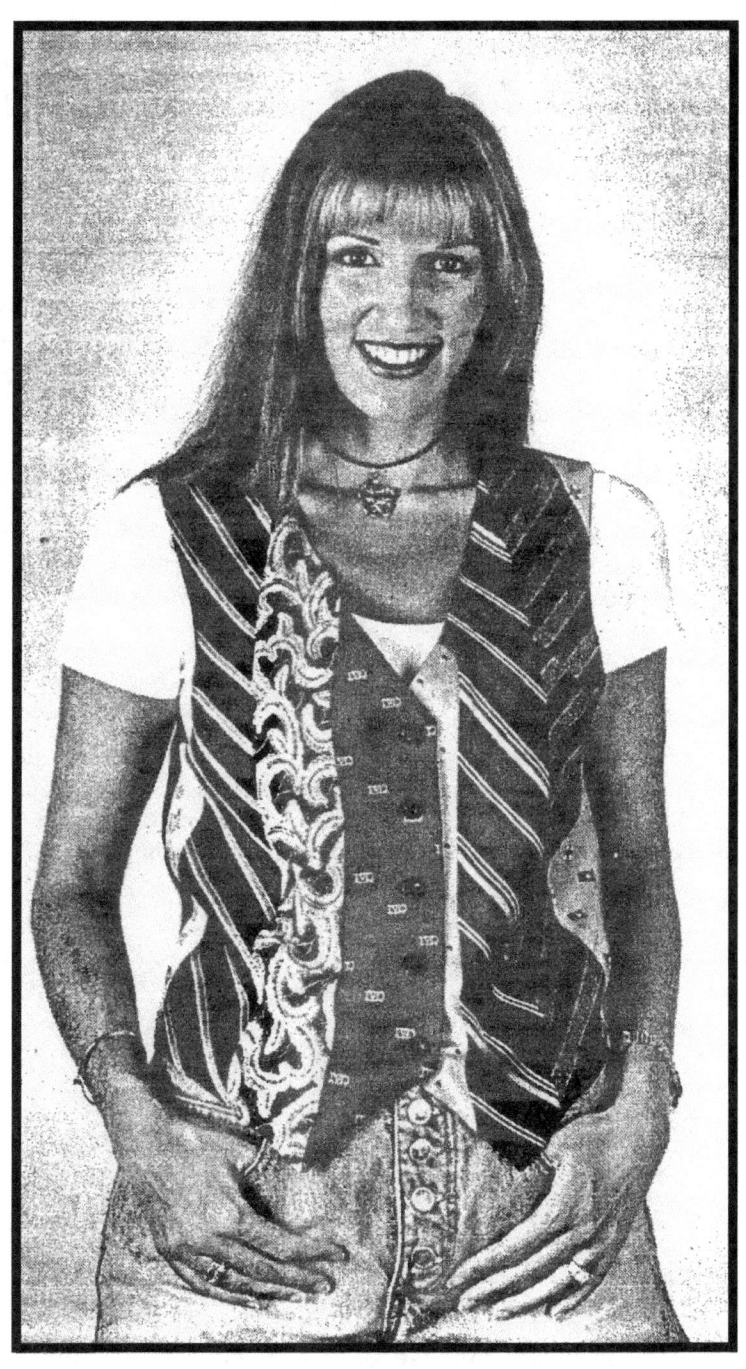

Model Patti Rao wears a Rose Weiss original vest, created from old silk ties. The Family Ties collection includes vests, jackets, and handbags.

153

A mother's story

Son with cerebral palsy inspires Naples resident to write a book

By Beth Francis
Staff Writer

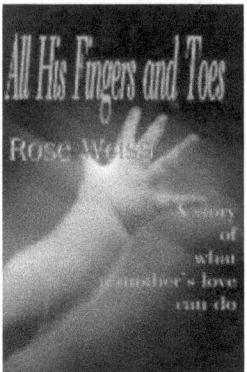

The first words Rose Weiss heard when her son was born were, "He's not breathing."

The doctor revived the tiny baby boy, but Weiss couldn't help but be concerned.

Ever optimistic, she tried to console herself. When the doctor came back into her room that evening on Sept. 8, 1938, and told her there may be a problem with her son, Weiss hopefully replied, "as long as he has all his fingers and toes."

As it turned out, Weiss' son had cerebral palsy, a term that refers to a broad range of chronic conditions that affect muscle control and brain functioning, resulting in physical and mental disabilities. A large number of factors can injure an infant's developing brain, both before and after birth. One of the biggest can be an insufficient amount of oxygen reaching the fetal or newborn brain.

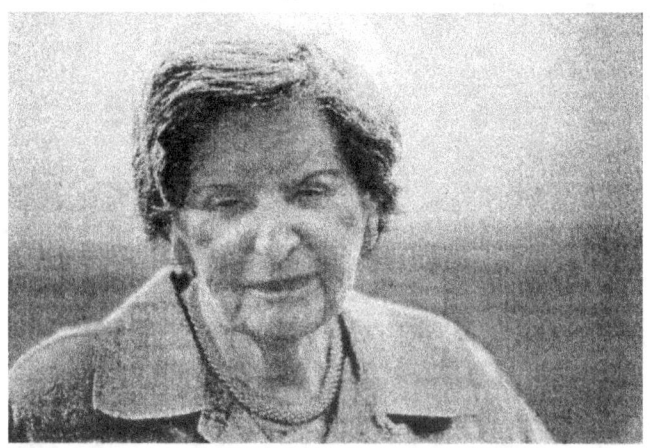

**Naples resident Rose Weiss tells the story of her son,
Elliott, who has cerebral palsy, in "All His Fingers and Toes."**
Matthew Ratajczak/Staff

154

Mom writes of work with disabled son

87-year-old wants others to benefit

By Jennifer Booth Reed

The News-Press

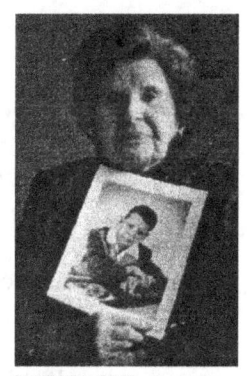

CLINT KRAUSE/The News-Press

North Naples – Rose Weiss waited 20 years to tell her story.

Now, at 87, she has published a book, detailing her struggles raising a son with cerebral palsy in the 1930s – before doctors fully understood the disorder and well before the days of state and federal laws protecting the disabled.

Today, she'll sign copies of her book, "All His Fingers and Toes: A story of what a mother's love can do," at Barnes & Noble in Naples.

Weiss, who moved from Miami to North Naples a year ago, first had an abbreviated form of her manuscript published in the Miami Herald in 1980.

With the encouragement of her daughter, Marlene, a North Naples architect and interior designer, Weiss expanded the story, revised it and looked for a publisher. She was rejected by the traditional publishing houses – although the company that puts out the "Chicken Soup for the Soul" series almost took it – and instead turned to the Internet.

Weiss' book is published through iUniverse.com, a subsidiary of Barnes & Noble that, for a price, will print books for aspiring authors. It cost her $135 to publish her book.

It's not a perfect system – authors do all of their corrections online and never meet their editors, and the book is rife with typographical errors.

But for Weiss, the venue didn't matter. She wants her story to inspire other parents who have disabled children.

"I feel I've attained the goal I've tried to reach – that all parents of cerebral palsy children know they're not alone," Weiss said.

Cerebral palsy is a chronic muscle condition that impacts body movement and muscle coordination. Those who have it may have muscle spasms and impaired mobility.

They may also have sight, hearing and speech problems, seizures and mental retardation.

Weiss' daughters said the book is among countless things her mother has done to help people with disabilities.

"Her whole life has been to help people with cerebral palsy," Marlene Weiss said. Rose and Eddie Weiss' son Elliott was born at home, delivered by a small-town family doctor in 1938.

Weiss believes a pill the doctor gave her to speed up her delivery may have caused complications. Elliott wasn't breathing at birth, and Weiss believes that the lack of oxygen to his brain may have resulted in cerebral palsy.

But she never got any answers.

L'Chaim

DECEMBER 25, 2007 • 16 TEVET, 5768

Jewish Journal

Moment in time

Museum photos include 1971 special needs b'nai mitzvah

By Sergio Carmona
JOURNAL STAFF WRITER

Naples resident Marlene Weiss caught a bit of family history at the

Jewish Museum of Florida.

The museum's permanent collection includes a picture of Rabbi Solomon Schiff, a long-time community leader, officiating a b'nai mitzvah for

cont.

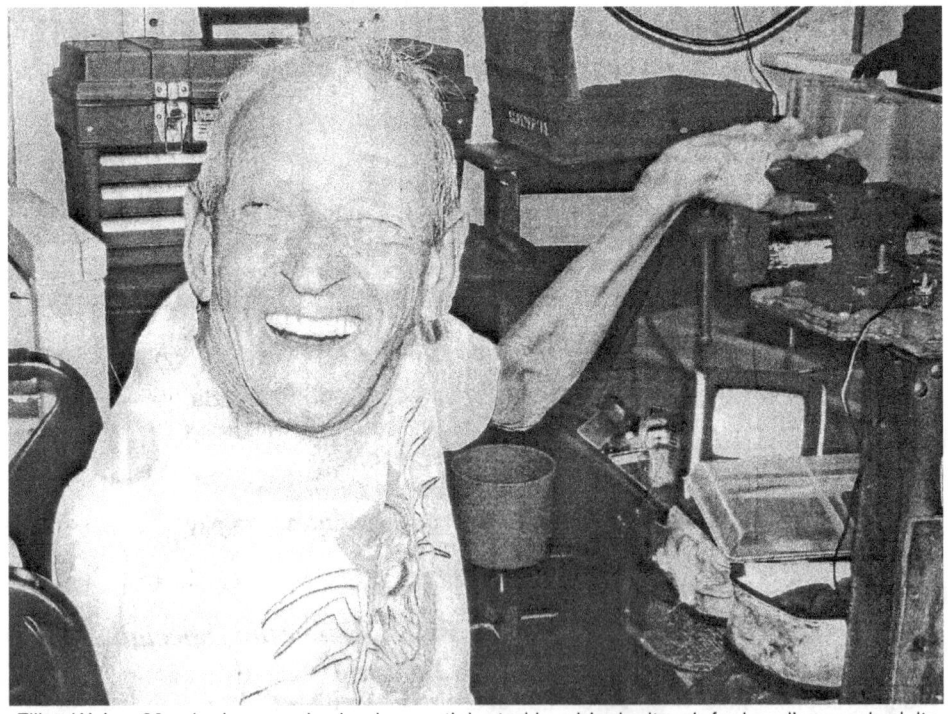

Elliott Weiss, 69, who has cerebral palsy, participated in a b'nai mitzvah for handicapped adults that was officiated by Rabbi Solomon Schiff in 1971. A photograph of that event is part of the Jewish Museum of Florida's permanent collection. Staff photo/Janeris Paredes handicapped adults May 10, 1971 at the Sunland Training Center in Miami, which closed in 2005. One of the celebrants in the photo is Marlene Weiss' older brother, Elliott, now 69. He was 33 at the time.

"I was very emotional that they would think enough to put the picture in the permanent collection of the Jewish Museum, and that a rabbi would think to go to a place where there's handicapped men [for the celebration]," said Marlene, now 56.

Elliott was diagnosed with cerebral palsy as a young child and currently resides at Woodhouse Cerebral Palsy Adult Home in Dania. His late mother, Rose Weiss, wrote a book called "All His Fingers and Toes: A Story of What a Mother's Love Can Do." The book mentions that the men in Sunland had a feeling of inadequacy because they could not have a bar mitzvah and they're Jewish.

"He knows he's Jewish, and I think that's important for him," Marlene said. "It's important for normal people. It's important for him."

Schiff came up with the idea to arrange a bar mitzvah. He said it was one of the more emotional experiences in all his years as a rabbi.

"I saw them bar mitzvahed with their parents and siblings, and they were in tears," he said. "The clients were able to say to older brothers, 'See, I was bar mitzvahed.'"

cont.

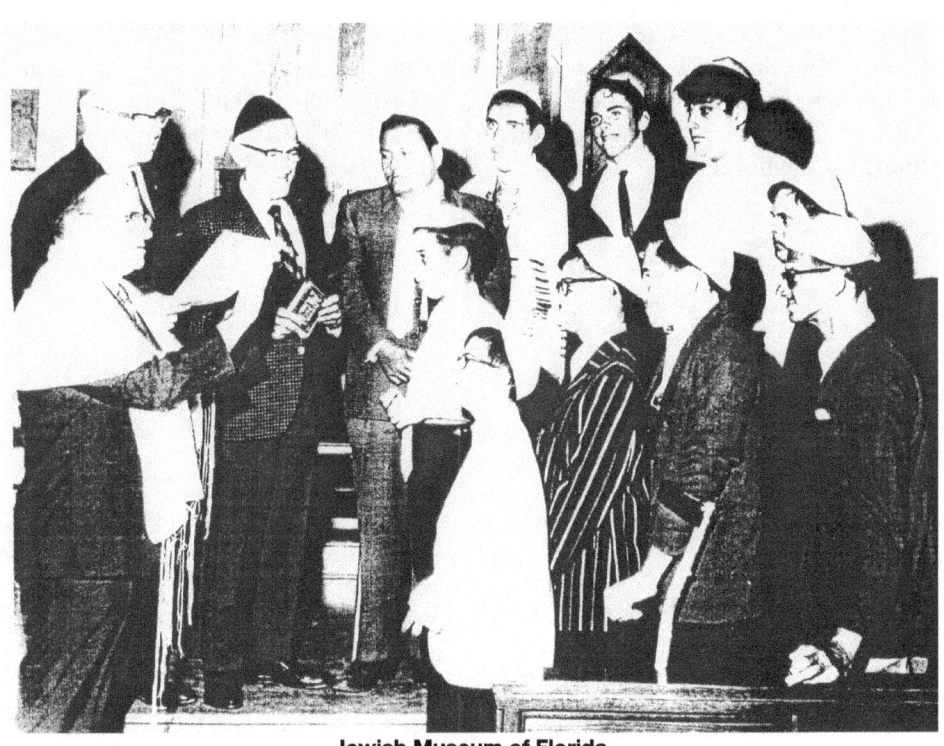

Jewish Museum of Florida
301 Washington Avenue, Miami Beach, Florida 33139-6965
Phone: 305-672-5044 Fax: 305-672-5933 www.jewishmuseum.com

Elliott said it was a great moment.

"It felt great," he said. "My mom and dad were there. And my cousins made a [film]."

When Elliott was born Sept. 8, 1938 in California, the doctors told Rose "he is not breathing," and had to breathe air into Elliott's lips until he finally breathed on his own. After the family took Elliott home, he was unable to eat and had to be fed with an eye-dropper and had trouble sitting and speaking. After several trips to a doctor in Pittsburgh, he was diagnosed with cerebral palsy. The family moved to Florida to enroll Elliott in a facility in Pompano Beach, where he learned to walk and talk. Learning disabilities prevented him from getting past fourth grade, and he was moved to a state facility in Gainesville, then to Fort Myers, then to Sunland. Marlene was born when Elliott was 12 and said he was only home for the holidays.

"It's like I grew up as an only child," she said. "It wasn't until I was older and my mom would go to Sunland on the weekend that I would go with her, or my parents would go to Fort Myers, so it was like I had a sibling that I didn't know."

Marlene is amazed that Elliott is able to use a computer, paints, and has a positive outlook and caring personality, as well as calling her every day to say, "Hello sweetheart, how are you?"

"I think that he's just a warm, caring person, that my mother put a lot into him and he loves family," she said. "We have a lot of cousins and the only thing he cares about is seeing his family."

For more information about the Jewish Museum of Florida, visit http://jewishmuseum.com/ or call 305-672-5044. The museum is located at 301 Washington Ave., Miami Beach.